The Reiki Master & Teacher New Awakening Sys

This Home Study Multimedia Course Teaches U
The Reiki Masters Sacred Symbol as used in all Reiki Attunements
How to Teach Reiki and Transfer the Spiritual Attunements

Home Study Multimedia Learning Material available for this Course
Course Book Manual and Tutorial Audio Course CD set
Free Healing Treatment Tutorials and Self Attunement Videos

"Welcome to your complete multimedia home study course.
I wish you every success in every area of your life"

Robert Bourne
Reiki Master Teacher

Naturally You
Publishing

United Kingdom

The Reiki Master-Teacher Manual

ISBN 978-0-9561159-2-8

A catalogue of this publication is available from the British Library

Naturally You Publishing

Published by Naturally You Publishing
All multimedia courses are distributed by Naturally You

For the latest information on
Spirituality, Healing and Sports Psychology please visit our website

www.naturallyyou.co.uk

'Naturally You' spiritual books and 'New Awakening' home study courses are available through Amazon booksellers and all main bookstores. New Awakening distributes our full range of multimedia home study courses. Visit our website at **www.new-awakening.co.uk**

'Naturally You Publishers' also supply a range of sports psychology interactive home study courses. These 'Into the Zone' mind coaching interactive courses are available for golf, snooker and other popular sports. Visit our website at **www.into-thezone.co.uk**

Table of Contents

Introduction and Background

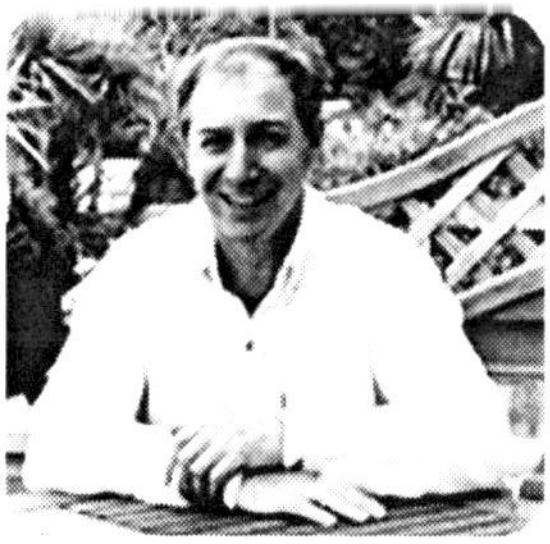

New Awakening

Love Healing & Wisdom

Spiritual Courses for your Development and Enlightenment

We are delighted to share with you our 'New-Awakening' courses to bring about your Personal Development and Spiritual Enlightenment. This complete healing experience enables absolute understanding of the mind body and spirit connection. Study all the courses in the five stages to achieve amazing results. Many students have accomplished in one year what would normally take 10 to 20 years of practice to achieve! The secret to this phenomenal growth is in the combination of Divine Reiki healing with an ancient eastern mystical wisdom philosophy as practiced by Dr Usui himself. The courses link together holistically and are expressed in logical, understandable everyday language, offering a total healing experience that will transform your life into a new experience of inner richness and enjoyable connectedness to the world around you. This truly is a revolutionary inner awakening approach, based on the source of creation – Unconditional Love.

The first stage of your development will establish an emotionally secure positive personality centred in love, able to heal and with the ability to create your own chosen destiny. To build this solid foundation three courses have been selected: The 'New Awakening Reiki Healing First Degree' will teach you how to heal yourself, friends, pets and plants through channelling the purity of the Reiki Universal Life Energy. Emotional healing is achieved through 'Love and Relationships' enabling you to discover the real meaning of intimacy and the secret of creating loving positive relationships centred in Unconditional Love. 'The Excellent You' will establish positive communication with an understanding of how your mind works in conjunction with the Law of Attraction, teaching you whole mind awareness meditation and creating abundance.

The second stage is achieved by helping others overcome their personal suffering through the magic of 'New Awakening Reiki Healing Second Degree' which deepens your Reiki and teaches you how to send healing long distances without having any physical contact. The training includes free energy attunements available from our website, which empower the student to use the Reiki symbols and their mantras. 'New Awakening' Spiritual Reiki will also attune you to the three spiritual bodies, not previously taught on the Reiki Second Degree course; you will have a direct spiritual experience of the three energies. The heart goes public and service work becomes part of your life.

In the third stage you will receive the 'New Awakening Reiki Master Degree Attunement'. In studying Dr Usui's personal spiritual practice contained in 'The Gateway to Enlightenment' you will learn how to transform your own personal mind's conditioning and belief systems into the true workings of the universal mind; how to establish 'Divine Wisdom'.

When you practice this system of healing as a tool for personal and spiritual development you will discover first hand that you are supported and guided by a kind and loving universe that will enable you to face all of the modern day challenges that you experience in your daily life.

"I would like to take this opportunity to send you my heartfelt appreciation and encouragement for the great courage that you have shown in embracing and expanding your life. I wish you every success in every area of your life from the bottom of my heart." Robert

The Reiki Master Attunement opens the life condition of Oneness

Everything in the universe is composed of energy. When you receive your Reiki Master attunement it is like plugging directly into the universal current of Unconditional Love. The source within you is in direct contact with the universal source that has no limits. There are no barriers to what this energy can do because it is the emotional expression of Divine Unconditional Love, an opening to the blissful state of Oneness. This is now a time of self-realising that you wish everyone to experience the same state of awareness as yourself. The only gift you can do for others is to give them attunements to the Divine; to awaken them to the same beauty that you are now experiencing. You know that through only sharing the same awareness together in this world, the same elevated consciousness, are we able to play, to dance and to create with each other, with the qualities of harmony, love and wisdom.

We are the ones to put barriers on the energy by our thoughts and soul's life consciousness. In Sharon's story after she had trustfully followed the New Awakening system, by working through the first four spiritual openings together with the study of the Seekers Guide, when she arrived at and experienced the Reiki Master's energy attunement she had the most beautiful Oneness experience possible. This experience happened naturally just like the petals of a flower opening when the sun shines its life giving warmth upon it. Sharon experienced that everything outside of her was just aspects of herself. She knew, from the inside, that she could change anything just by her desire to do so; she had realised the Oneness of life. Even her relationships changed automatically in a beautiful loving way; her boyfriend, who had been previously non-committal for many years, just had an experience of love when Sharon had her attunement and spontaneously without thought proposed to her.

'New Awakening' - About the Spiritual System

Enlightenment throughout the ages is always the same, when a human being awakens to the inner realm of the mystic law of creation. These great personal experiences have been translated into many religious, spiritual and mystical practices that have been taught over many centuries to help society. We have tremendous respect and appreciation for all past different teaching methods because they have brought us spiritually to where we are today.

This is a very exciting time as there is the emergence of a new energy consciousness occurring throughout the world. What is happening is that many of these teachings are now transforming into a direct spiritual experience. There are many individuals who are now awakening to an inner Divine wisdom resulting in a tremendous love and compassion for themselves, humanity and the natural environment. You could say that the seeds of the old spiritual teachings are now transforming; they are now starting to flower within society.

We understand this as a shift in consciousness that is starting to take place on the earth today; the start of a new golden, human-spiritual era for all of mankind to experience. There have been many prophesies which support that this change in consciousness will be happening at this time. The main shift that is taking place in society today is the change in the way that enlightenment is now being experienced.

Throughout mankind's history we have had the experience of isolated individuals achieving enlightenment, teaching disciples who in turn have left teachings and spiritual practices for us to follow. These teachings and practices have been left to help us understand our relationship with the creative source of existence. What we are seeing happen today is quite the opposite whereby personal enlightenment is now being experienced by many individuals. This phenomenon is now slowly spreading throughout the whole of society as each enlightened individual influences others to do the same.

Having had the privilege of this direct Divine experience, the founder of the 'New Awakening' system, Robert Bourne, being aware of this new phenomenon has been divinely guided to create a modern system of spiritual awakening that is appropriate for today's age. This new system enables the individual to have a direct experience of the laws of creation; eventually resulting in personal enlightenment. When you experience this new system of learning in its entirety a new spiritual awakening becomes possible.

The new awakening system, created for modern day living, consists of a series of personal and spiritual development Awakening Teachings plus the four Reiki stages of learning. The Reiki stages of learning contain the traditional Reiki attunements which I am offering to everyone free of charge as my gift to mankind, learning concepts plus additional wisdom practices at each stage of development. These additional teachings provide spiritual experiences that become personal foundations, building blocks for the individual's next stage of spiritual evolution. All the four stages of Reiki interlink into one complete 'New Awakening' personal enlightenment system for the student.

The 'New Awakening' system fundamentally differs from the traditional workshop as it offers the student a direct inner spiritual experience of the teaching that they are learning. As you study this spiritual guide you will receive a 'Spiritual Awakening Transfer', guided from Unconditional Love. This will awaken a direct inner experience and realization for you.

The Unconditional Love energy transfers are contained within these teachings and are provided without charge on my videos. They will attune your chakra system to bring about your spiritual realization of the teaching you are learning; a new awakening with a change in consciousness occurs as a result.

These 'New Awakening' Courses and Workshops will create a successful individual with a compassionate heart. You will have the ability to create your own reality, free from the conditioning and limitations of the self. They will awaken you to your own healing; to your own inner state of Unconditional Love and most importantly to your inner teacher providing you with Divine Wisdom in each moment of your existence. You will learn the workings of human spiritual life within all aspects of your relationships and your personal experience of daily life.

A New Awakening spiritual teacher becomes an automatic experience. This is not based upon attendance of the training course but is based upon the ability to channel Unconditional Love from the crown chakra. 'New Awakening' spiritual teachers will have to evolve to a state of 'Being' that resonates with Unconditional Love, not just attend a training course and collect a certificate; otherwise they will be unable to transfer Divine Wisdom and awaken the spiritual teachings within those they wish to help.

The 'New Awakening Spiritual System' consists of Five Stages of Development with Seven Spiritual Openings

The 'New Awakening' system has been designed and created from Divine spiritual guidance. The New Awakening system understands that if the student has not opened themselves spiritually at the foundation awakening energy stages of their development, they will be unable to progress to the next awakening stage. This is true even if they have previously undertaken the assumed required training. The truth is that you are one with the Divine, although you may be blocked off from this direct connection with the illusionary beliefs you hold within your soul and mind body. This system gently guides you to unlock this beautiful birthright connection to enable your life to flourish into the amazing person you really are. It is for this reason I have released the secret formula to unlock this mystical Divine connection directly for you. Through following the attunement initiation that I will give you free of charge, you will discover how to reconnect yourself to that which is hidden within you. Yes you do it to yourself; I am just your guide. Beware of anyone who tells you that this is not possible. The very idea is charged with illusion, power and control.

Through releasing the secret to the attunement process I have gone against the need to have another perform the ceremony for you. I have broken the tradition which has been passed down over many years. The reason for doing this is two fold. Over several years the awareness that I have been enlightened to has guided me to release this method of self spiritual attunement to anyone who wishes to experience it. The other reason is that the time is right now for as many people as possible to awaken into their spiritual body. For many lifetimes I have taught these teachings in the traditional way, now is the culmination of my soul's mission to share this directly with you in a new direct way.

All the teachings and stages of development that make up this system have been proven by many students who have verified the tremendous depth of beauty and simplicity of the whole process. You are now in a privileged position to enjoy what others have taken many years to experience by having a direct sharing of the Masters' secrets.

There is one fact that I would like to share with you which is in respect to the level of effectiveness a spiritual attunement will have upon you. Anyone who offers you any form of teaching or spiritual experience can only help you arrive at the same level of consciousness that they themselves have obtained. Choose your teacher with great care. Over the last few years I have been involved in the world of Reiki. I have been surprised as to how watered down the teachings have become. This is not a criticism of the teachers of Reiki but as a result of my direct experience. I have met many teachers who did not have any spiritual understanding as to what they are trying to transmit, even teachers who had no faith in Reiki at all! The angelic realm of the Divine will always come forward to make a connection with anyone who desires their presence, so even the students of these teachers will have received great benefit.

The problem with the distortion that has been introduced into this system is a result of the illusions held within the mind of some modern Reiki Masters who, as a result have watered down, complicated and distorted the beauty of this natural healing comforter. It is for this reason that I have released directly to mankind the truth, as far as I have experienced it. I promise you that all of my students have grown in consciousness and those who have been re-attuned by me from other disciplines have experienced a much deeper meaningful spiritual energy experience as a result.

The other concern is that people who try and connect directly with the source of Unconditional Love, through by-passing the spiritual foundation training, can awaken their repressed, negative pain body of illusion within their soul. When this happens they can fall into fear, withdrawing from their spiritual self, finding they are unable to cope with their new experience. This dark night of the soul experience can be avoided! The only solution for this person is to go back and work through the stages of spiritual energy opening again. We have discovered that many training courses are purely theoretical and the teachings have never been transformed into personal spiritual experiences; the energy then stays within the mind of the student.

When a spiritual foundation and pathway has been established in the energy system and soul of the student the next doorway can then open; this awakening automatically happens with the 'New Awakening' training. All life experiences will then be met at the soul level with healing, transforming into love and balance.

This also explains why people get stuck on their spiritual journey. For example even though someone may have received the Reiki Masters Attunement or a Oneness attunement, if a foundation stage is by-passed, or the chakra energy system has not fully opened, the student will not be able to fully awaken to the next stage of development. This is controlled by the natural law of life. In this example the enlightenment of the Reiki Master's heart chakra will not fully open and be personally experienced if the three energy bodies have not been awakened at the Reiki Second Degree stage of spiritual awakening. Enlightenment just 'IS' - you are unable to buy it - you have to awaken to it.

The 'New Awakening' method has a compassionate methodical approach through providing proven energy experiences which build upon each other creating a solid safe foundation for the student. This compassionate system created for the individual will enable the next spiritual opening to naturally occur safely. 'New Awakening' will support you with Divine Wisdom, Healing and Unconditional Love.

The 'New Awakening' system also provides three wisdom based companion personal and spiritual home study courses, with tutorial CDs, to support the seven spiritual openings. These courses are contained within the book and seven CD set 'The Seekers Guide for a New Awakening' and the courses are 'The Excellent You, 'Love and Relationships' and 'The Gateway to Enlightenment'.

When the CDs are listened to repeatedly, they have a transformative effect upon the consciousness of the listener. The 'Ah Ha' moments just keep coming over and over again. What could not be understood through reading alone becomes an enlightenment experience as the change in consciousness occurs at the soul level of awareness within you.

When you clear the blocks, transform your illusions you naturally awaken to your own Divinity. Great spiritual teachers who have spontaneously awakened to their true nature, like Eckhart Tolle, try to encourage us that this natural Divine state of being is really here 'in the now' and that we are just veiled or blocked off from it by the illusions within our own mind. The students who have studied all three 'New Awakening' courses contained within 'The Seekers Guide for a New Awakening' have accelerated their spiritual development. Enlightenment 'IS' 'here and now', it is our illusions and misguided beliefs held in our karmic soul body that prevent us from having it all – right now! The courses will provide you with a wisdom foundation at your soul level to prepare you to have this birthright experience of Enlightenment.

To achieve the beautiful experience of personal enlightenment we have discovered that the following foundation spiritual gates, when opened within you in the following order, provide a gentle soul transition for this beautiful experience to occur:

First Spiritual Opening: The free attunement to Reiki Universal Life Healing Energy as experienced in Reiki First Degree. This opens the heart chakra and the individual begins their spiritual journey; they are on the pathway to direct enlightenment. It is advisable to study the Reiki course manual and follow the exercises contained on the tutorial CDs. The home study of the three 'New Awakening' companion courses contained in 'The Seekers Guide', is now introduced to you to assist your spiritual learning experience.

Second and Third Spiritual Openings: This is the attunement and awakening to the energy of the present, the power symbol for physical healing with its complementary emotional symbol of Love Sei-Hei-Ki. The second and third spiritual openings are experienced within part one of the Reiki Second Degree course manual together with the free Reiki 2nd degree spiritual self-attunements. These two symbols form the base two parts of a triangle and when opened allow the soul to soul connection to occur in a more powerful way through the crown chakra as described in stage three. The base chakra is grounded with the power symbol Cho-Ku-Rei as it brings Divinity into 'the present' the material expression of daily life. The heart chakra, the cross-roads of the lower and higher self, is directly connected to Unconditional Love through the emotional symbol; providing greater love and compassion to be experienced.

Fourth Spiritual Opening: The attunement to the distant healing symbol Hon-Sha-Ze-Sho-Nen. This happens through the crown chakra directly through the Divine chakra. 'The divinity in me meets the divinity in you'. This enables the Divine spiritual healing experience directly from soul to soul to occur. This explains the awareness of white light with the out of body experience reported by many of our students. This fourth spiritual opening is experienced within the Reiki Second Degree course manual and through following the guidance contained on the tutorial CDs.

Fifth and Sixth Spiritual Openings: The attunement to Reiki Masters energy, Dai-Ko-Myo. When the spiritual openings one to four have been established the heart chakra of the student can now fully open, radiating Unconditional Love for all of mankind. It is at this stage that 'New Awakening' differs from most Reiki methods used in the West as it includes an additional attunement to Divine Wisdom. This awakens the higher self within the third eye chakra of the student. This connection accesses the Divine Laws of creation enabling life choices to be made with Divine Wisdom, as opposed to personal intuition. This transforms illusion into enlightenment.

Seventh Spiritual Opening: This self attunement completes the journey of the soul by ascending to the crown chakra. The heart chakra compassionately radiates the Reiki Master Energy, the soul transcends to the crown with the higher self moving down from the crown to reside in the third eye. Healing and Wisdom now combine being expressed as the Unconditional Love of the Source of creation. This is the stage of mysticism, of becoming. Life becomes the experience of bliss, wisdom and Oneness with all existence. The individual moves beyond religious, race, national prejudice, written teachings or dogma. It is at this stage that the 'New Awakening' spiritual teacher is born.

Traditional Courses Versus New Awakening Courses

The Universal Life Healing Energy has been traditionally taught in three stages known as the Reiki First Degree, Reiki Second Degree and Reiki Master/Teacher. The students are usually required to take their own notes, or are provided with a basic course manual, at the workshop. Traditionally, Reiki has been taught in the West orally. This means that the student has to remember what the teacher is saying which can cause some stress. This system can create the possibility of the 'Chinese Whispers' syndrome whereby information changes or becomes distorted.

In contrast, the New Awakening system has addressed this problem by providing the student with fully comprehensive multimedia learning material thereby negating the necessity to take notes. This enables the New Awakening student to fully enter into the energy experiences contained within the manuals and through following the tutorial guides experienced on the interactive CDs. The attunements are provided free of charge and you can repeat them as often as you like.

New Awakening teaches The Universal Life Healing Energy in three stages; Reiki First Degree, Reiki Second Degree, Reiki Master/Reiki Master Teacher, with each stage consisting of two parts. The first part is the professional home study multimedia course learning material. The second part is the practical 'Self Attunement' energy experience, that is provided free of charge as our gift to you from our website. (www.new-awakening.co.uk)

The Story of Sharon

"After a good few years of enduring the usual life struggles, including ill health and relationship issues, my partner treated me to a much needed long weekend away at a health spa. This was where I had my first Reiki treatment. It was the most amazing experience of my life to date alongside child birth. I came away from the weekend knowing that I would be spending at least the next 6 months trying to work out what had actually happened to me.

In September 2007 I began my search on the internet reading various descriptions of Reiki, when I came across the New Awakening website. Robert described his study of many different forms of Reiki and had not limited himself to one style, as had other teachers. Having an engineering background, this appealed to me, as I am always looking for logic, reason and proof in what I learn.

Realising the need to understand the experiences of my first Reiki treatment, I plucked up the courage to call Robert. Shortly thereafter I received the Reiki First Degree course hand book through the post. I remember being told at that time, that if I did not want to experience change, then this was not the course for me. Sat here a few years later, I cannot believe how poignant those words now seem.

I spent the next few months reading through the course material in snippets of spare time, fitted between my young family, an engineering design job, running a house and maintaining a long distance relationship.

It was December 2007 when I met Robert and joined a couple of other students on the Reiki I course.

Reading through the material at home I had felt very comfortable with understanding the technicalities of a basic Reiki treatment. However, being on the course and actually feeling and experiencing the energies was quite something else. I felt I was now truly on the path to discovering what I had experienced in my first Reiki treatment.

Receiving my first attunement was like becoming aware of a whole new dimension to life which had been previously hidden from me. I remember feeling an amazing sense of inner peace but also being surrounded by bright and vivid colours.

The opportunity to give my first Reiki treatment in a caring and supportive environment gave me the courage to realise that this was something I could actually do. With a new radiant glow on my face and my First Reiki certificate in hand, I set off to increase my experience of this wonderful new dimension. I spent the next six weeks practicing my new found skills on myself, friends and family. The positive feedback I had from other people was amazing and I became a very popular person. At the same time I was also noticing many personal changes which were highlighted to me by using the 21 day journal.

As time progressed my confidence grew and with so many people around me now interested in Reiki, I decided to continue my studies and sent away for the Reiki II course. I also studied the additional courses 'The Excellent You' and 'Love and Relationships', both of which I still refer to today.

During the home study period of Reiki II, I found many questions answered. From the practical aspect of Reiki I had many experiences where I felt guided to certain positions without knowing why. All these experiences I now find were being described in this course. I was also conscious of the fact that in the past I had always struggled with the process of learning and with retention of information. However, I now realised a new ability and enthusiasm to learn. This spread into other areas of my life too.

At the beginning of March 2008, I attended the Reiki II course. Before arriving for this course I already felt very comfortable with giving Reiki treatments and with understanding the course material. I came away feeling I had reached a whole new level on my personal journey. I was amazed at the effect of experiencing the energies using alternative methods such as chanting and humming. During my Second Degree attunement, the colours visible to me became brighter. I came away feeling a great sense that there was a much longer journey ahead of me than I had first anticipated.

I went home and continued giving Reiki treatments and found that the basic principles of Reiki had now reached into every part of my life. I could see my own failings more clearly and began working on becoming a better person with a life of value and quality.

From the Second course I also returned with the 'Gateway to Enlightenment' manual. I spent the next six months reading and studying this book. This was a much more challenging text and included some new scientific ideologies for me, which I found very interesting. The proof of distance healing behind me placed me in a much better position to grasp these new realities. 'The Gateway to Enlightenment' currently lives by my bedside and a year on I can still pick it up and gain 'Ah Ha' moments.

To continue my journey, towards the end of 2008 I gave Robert a call to discuss continuing on to Masters Level. After a lengthy conversation and some time for me to think things through I concurrently booked the Masters and Master Teacher courses. Receiving the relevant manuals with only just a month to go before the practical I was not sure if I was going to be ready, but reading through the manuals made me realise that I had learnt a great deal from the Gateway to Enlightenment and I was definitely ready for this now. I was really looking forward to this course with no hesitation or doubt, a real change in character for me.

In January 2009, I was given the gift of the Masters attunement, which personally became my biggest and best step.

Through studying the Gateway to Enlightenment and the other accompanying courses, I gained many understandings with my mind which had a significant impact on my life as a whole as I became more understanding of people, emotions and reactions. I then began to find that life does not surprise you in a way that it did before. You start to see things much earlier giving you time to be better prepared, as opposed to living in a constant reactive style.

My Masters attunement really did bring all the teachings to life in a way that I could not have understood before. During the attunement itself, I was aware of many different faces joining my being; an experience for which I have no words.

The following morning I had the amazing experience of waking and finding I not only clearly remembered the dream I had that night, but I also understood it immediately with a deep sense of knowing. I then had the realisation that my mind had understood and learnt from the teachings but before the attunement my heart and soul had not understood these lessons and I felt a shift of the level of understanding to my subconscious.

Now I feel a connection not just between body and mind which comes from Reiki I and II, but also now the connection with the soul. The best way for describing this feeling is to imagine that it is a cold winter's night and you have had a good meal and you are wrapped up warm and comfortable in front of an open fire and are surrounded by all the people who are closest to you. This is the feeling which I now carry with me all the time and it is the most beautiful experience.

After the Masters followed the Master Teacher course which felt like a very natural progression.

I am now looking forward to teaching this beautiful system of healing for the self and others and will continue with Reiki healing for those that do not wish or are not yet ready to make the journey. I shall continue my personal study and self healing and look forward to an interesting and challenging future.

Life carries on but I am now able to deal with issues that arise with more speed and confidence. Having heightened intuition and plenty of new life skills enable you to recognise signs of approaching tests in your life. This whole process becomes apparent as you look back on your life. Occasionally I am able to see where it is going. However you're never quite sure how things are going to happen, so life remains full of surprises.

I would like to take this opportunity to offer my sincere thanks to Robert for his continuing support and his dedication to spread the understanding of Reiki and Spirituality to the Whole World".

Namaste Sharon Tucker

Home Study Plan of Action

How to Study this Multimedia Course Material

Preparation

1. Read this manual all the way through quickly to get the idea of what you are going to learn
2. Listen to the tutorial CDs (Optional)
3. Prepare your 21 day journal. Continue in your Reiki 2nd degree journal. Start day one of your journal when you receive your attunement to Master's Reiki healing; when you use the Attunement Video.

Practice – (Remember to record everything in your journal)

1. Attune yourself to Reiki Healing using the VIDEO provided – see below.
2. Practice drawing the symbol for The Reiki Master's healing until you know it by heart. Awaken the Master's healing energy of Dai-Ko-Myo using the chanting method explained on page 22.
3. Study pages 27 and 28 and then chant the mantra for 10 minutes with your eyes open.
4. This practice of chanting will directly connect you to the source of creation therefore whatever you desire will quickly be realised through the Law of Attraction. The whole philosophy of Ichinen Sanzen is inscribed on the Mandala Gohonzon on page 27. Chant with your eyes open and focused upon the Mandala to awaken your deepest Buddha Wisdom.
5. Repeatedly re-read this manual to reveal its layered meaning. You will discover that as your consciousness changes the teachings will reveal new meanings to you.
6. When the CDs are listened to repeatedly, they have a transformative effect upon the consciousness of the listener. The 'Ah Ha' moments just keep coming over and over again. What could not be understood through reading alone becomes an enlighten-

ment experience as the change in consciousness occurs at the soul level of awareness within you.

How to use the Distant Attunement Video

1. Watch the VIDEO all the way through on your own, in a place where you won't be interrupted, to get the gist of what is going to happen. Unplug the phone etc.
2. To feel a deeper experience continue by relaxing your state of mind by doing the Breathing Meditation listed at the back of this manual. This will prepare you to attune yourself more effectively.
3. Start your Reiki Healing and then start chanting Dai-Ko-Myo to invoke the Master's energy, as it is this energy that is used to transfer the spiritual attunements.
4. Then replay the Video again from the beginning, this time taking 3 deep breaths, centring your awareness in your sacral chakra, moving your energy down from your mind. Relax and close your eyes. Now imagine that it is you sitting in the chair receiving the attunement.
5. When instructions are given, this is when I will now be talking to you and guiding you through the attunement. Following the sequence you can either do the instructed actions physically or see yourself doing them in your imagination.

"Reading this book together with listening to the sound of my voice on the CDs will enable a Divine inner shift of consciousness to occur within you. I wish you tremendous happiness in every area of your life. May the mystic law help you create the life of your dreams as you become a blessing to mankind." Robert Bourne – New Awakening course creator.

The Reiki Master

Deepening your Reiki Experience with Master's Wisdom leads on to Teach Reiki

Welcome. I honour your decision to become a Reiki Master and I thank you for choosing me as your Master and teacher. It is an honour and one I value highly. By choosing me as your Master, we have created an unbreakable bond and I will always be there for you. This is not a guru/disciple relationship; it is, however, a lasting relationship formed by two equals, who support each other's endeavours.

Once you have obtained the Master level, you assume a larger responsibility for your life's actions. In order to teach Reiki and Divine wisdom you must live it; you must have absolute trust in Reiki's energy and the mystic law of life. You are now starting on your voyage to become a Reiki Master and Usui Reiki Teacher. You will soon receive the Master attunement and be given the Master symbol.

New Awakening Spiritual Teacher

The final stage of an individual's development is to ascend to the crown chakra. The Master's wisdom resides in the third eye chakra and is in fact 'The Mystic Law' of creation 'The Avatar'. I shall remind you of the seventh spiritual opening to occur within the New Awakening system of enlightenment.

Seventh Spiritual Opening: This attunement completes the journey of the soul by ascending to the crown chakra. The heart chakra compassionately radiates the Reiki Master Energy of Dai-Ko-Myo, the soul transcends to the crown with the higher self moving down from the crown to reside in the third eye. Healing and Wisdom now combine, being expressed as the Unconditional Love of the Source of creation. This is the stage of mysticism, of becoming. Life becomes the experience of bliss, wisdom and Oneness with all existence. The individual moves beyond religious, race and national prejudice. It is at this stage that the 'New Awakening' spiritual teacher is born.

The Divine manifests into all phenomena 'How the one becomes the many'

I would like to share a Vedic Yoga explanation of how the Divine manifests into existence. This concept is at the heart of the Eastern Mystical Teachings and is at the core of the teachings learnt on the New Awakening spiritual teacher course. The following five stages explain how the core of existence manifests into all phenomena, 'How the one becomes the many'.

1. The source of all things, of creation is 'Intelligent Pure Divine Consciousness, Bliss with the experience of Truth'.

2. As the supreme creator the Source manifests into all creation, the cosmos and the universe.

3. Unity Consciousness, Oneness Consciousness occurs where one Divine being is created which incarnates as an Avatar to guide us in the realm of duality.

4. This Divine being incarnates into everyone as the higher self to guide the process of creation which is carried out by the self. A creative relationship now exists between all of life and the Divine.

5. The female aspect of creation is in communion with the male aspect of creation and is celebrated. The human being, once awakened to this connection becomes 'The Avatar'.

The Reiki Master makes a Commitment to be in Service to Others

A Master healer requires the following four qualities: trust, faith, love and humility. As a Reiki Master you are now the pathway of the healing energy called Source. In order to effectively function as the guardian of such tremendous energy, you must have absolute trust in the Reiki healing power as well as the faith that you are capable of working with and teaching others how to do likewise.

Although different healers may channel the energy by a variety of different methods, none can teach or heal without compassionate love and humility. You must learn to love and accept the hardest person in the world to love - yourself. There is no ego in using or teaching Reiki. This aspect will be easier for you as you will have had the benefit of understanding and practicing the universal mind laws of Divine Wisdom.

You are the co-creator of the healing process, allowing the Source within to join the Source without and exist through you, thereby balancing all it comes in contact with.

The Master is an Inner Experience of Divine Connection that Becomes Eternally Indestructible

Congratulations. I know that you are ready for this transition and I offer my deepest heartfelt support but in reality you are now one with the Source.

The teacher is within and you will be connected to the consciousness of The Ascendant Masters and will continue learning from your direct connection with enlightened beings.

I wish to remind you of the key points of this beautiful state of existence. You will experience the Bliss Body of the Divine; Pure Unconditional Loving Presence. It is from this union that:

1. Unconditional love and healing flow eternally from your heart chakra
2. Universal wisdom is accessed in each moment of existence
3. Unconditional Love, Healing and Divine Wisdom automatically become available for the benefit of others without effort

These Three Aspects Become One

Unity Consciousness

NASA astronaut Dr. Edgar Mitchell came to this conclusion on his return trip from space: "In one moment I realised that this universe is intelligent. It is proceeding in a direction and we have something to do with that direction. And that creative spirit, the creative intent that has been the history of the planet, comes from within us and it is out there – it is all the same …….

Consciousness itself is what is fundamental and energy-matter is the product of consciousness .... If we change our heads about who we are and can see ourselves as creative, eternal beings creating physical experience, joined at that level of existence we call consciousness, then we start to see and create this world that we live in quite differently."

The Third Degree Reiki for Personal Growth and Service

The Third Degree Reiki attunement and symbol take you further on your journey of growth and expansion. As more light becomes your life, you share this light with others automatically. The more you share this light the more light enters your being. It is as if you have now entered into a win-win situation; the more light you give the more light you receive.

Your life path is accelerated and supported by the totality of the Reiki energy. In a way, there is more work to do in the sense of letting go and taking on new challenges, however we access more guidance supported by a kind and loving universe with the help of the Master symbol and the Master's energy.

The Heart Centre is the main focus of the third-degree attunement. We unfold in love as we blossom in our unique way dancing with the benevolent forces of the universe, to the music of our life force. When you are ready many obstacles melt and frontiers disappear. Every moment can become an opportunity to express light as kindness towards oneself and towards all others.

Wrapped in the loving blessing of Reiki we might find the path steeper sometimes, but also easier, as we take on more responsibility and learn to love more.

You are ready, you are love. Live that love more and more every moment of your life in all the little things of daily life. Remember Light and Reiki is with you - always.

The Master's Level of Consciousness

All problems are solved and dissolve by entering into a level of existence where no problem exists. (Beyond Karma – beyond confrontation). Sitting on the Lotus flower.

A problem is solved not by confrontation but through going to a level of consciousness where no problem exists! Unity consciousness – The Oneness of life – Unconditional Love.

Becoming Non Change in the Face of Constant Change is 'The Master'

DAI KO MYO

The Reiki Master's Symbol

Dai-Ko-Myo is the Reiki Master Empowerment Symbol. It is the fourth symbol used by Dr. Usui and represents enlightenment.

Dai-Ko-Myo lifts us to a higher plane of consciousness and is said to heal at the level of soul or at the level of the spiritual body.

Dai-Ko-Myo is the key which accesses the full potential of Reiki in its totality.

Dai - means Great;
Dai - used here represents an enlightened great man.

Ko - means light. Ko is a picture of a man holding fire over the top of his head and running or moving forward. This signifies to pass the energy to others, the torch carrier, also light, expansion or radiance at the Crown Chakra.

Myo – means to open and reveal the essential nature of the mystic law. Myo means that your subtle healing body will have a radiance brighter than the sun and moon.

Dai-Ko-Myo can also be translated as 'Great Enlightenment'.

My interpretation is: 'The Reiki Master is the torch bearer to transfer and awaken the Divine light inside the heart of the individual, the transfer of the great fire of the Divine, the comforter and healer. This can be seen to be the transfer of 'The Holy Ghost'.

Evoking 'The Masters Symbol'

Chant this Mantra until you become one with its energy

1. Draw the symbol three times and chant the mantra for as long as you require, enabling you to feel the powerful Reiki energy manifesting in your whole being; until you become one with the energy.

2. You can stop chanting as soon as you can feel the energy in your body - this could be for a period of ten minutes up to one-hour duration.

3. As soon as you are completely happy you are one with the energy, stop chanting, close your eyes and enjoy the experience. Go into it; merge yourself with the feelings and sensations of being one with Dai-Ko-Myo.

4. It is good to deepen your experience with Dai-Ko-Myo by repeating this exercise every day for at least three days.

Uses of the Symbol

- This symbol can now be used for your own empowerment and connection with the Divine energy of Reiki.

- The more you use Dai-Ko-Myo the more you will expand your own consciousness into the state of Enlightenment.

- It can also be used in all healings, distance and hands-on, private healing and when you are healing others.

- This symbol is used for initiations and attunements of the Reiki degrees in others.

DAI KO MYO   Great Enlightenment

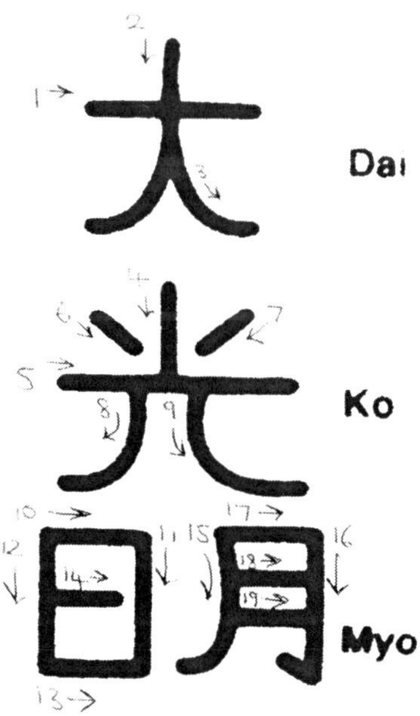

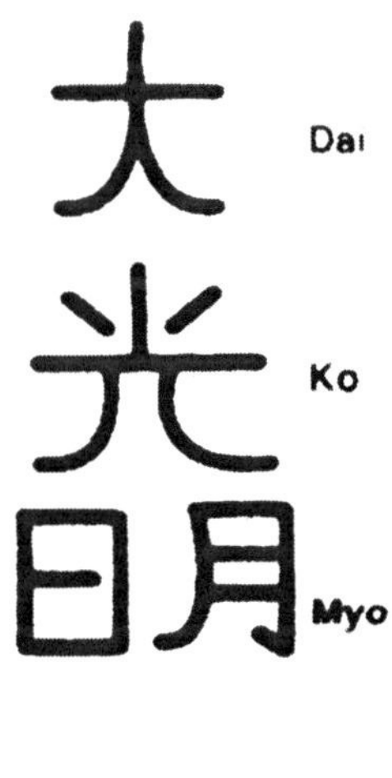

The Lotus Sutra - Masters Wisdom

Dr Usui - The Founder of Reiki Healing

The Buddhist Wisdom Sutra not taught in Reiki Healing

Dr Usui's original quest was in search of his personal enlightenment. His enlightenment can be attributed to establishing a foundation, a pathway within his soul by embracing the correct Buddhist Wisdom teaching. To discover the true story and history of Dr Usui's life established Reiki organizations have recently discovered that the fundamental practice that he embraced, before his enlightenment, was with the Buddhist sect known as The Tendai school of Buddhism. I am most grateful to them for their research because this explains to me that the cause for Dr Usui's fusion with the Divine, the establishment of unity consciousness can be attributed to his practice of 'The Lotus Sutra'.

Over the last 20 years I have been most fortunate to have studied and practiced in depth numerous Buddhist philosophies among which was 'The Lotus Sutra'. This was also the cause for my own enlightenment, my fusion with the Divine and the establishment of the wisdom body within my own life. I was aware that an aspect for personal enlightenment was lacking within the Reiki training syllabus. This aspect is the wisdom body philosophy which is the cause for enlightenment.

The traditional Reiki training teaches the effects of Dr Usui's enlightenment, the flowering of the Divine heart. This is Reiki as taught and practiced today. It was approximately fifteen years ago when I experienced a fusion with the Divine Beloved Universal Consciousness. My only desire at that time was to share the unconditional love, healing and wisdom with the whole world. I quickly learned that the life condition, the presence of the Divine was far too powerful to be experienced directly by most people. This enormous life condition was the effect, the flowering of Divine presence.

I have patiently waited for the right time to be able to share my experience with others. I was guided to study Reiki healing in 2003 and through my training it became apparent to me that no wisdom philosophy was being taught within the Reiki syllabus. The year was 2004 and thanks to the endeavours of William Lee Rand, Frank Arjava Petter and Walter Lubeck a much fuller picture of the true story behind Mikao Usui and the history of Reiki have now been established. It is from this new research that it has been established that Dr Usui studied in a Tendai Buddhist school and practiced meditation of the Lotus Sutra.

It is this mystical profound teaching that I have included in this course so that you too can experience the awakening of Divine Wisdom. First of all I will give you a little history about the Tendai School and its relationship to 'The Lotus Sutra'.

The Tendai School

A school founded by Dengyo in Japan. Its head Temple is Enryakuji on Mount Hiei. In 804 Dengyo made the journey to T'ang China, where he completed the study of the T'ien-t'ai teachings. He returned to Japan in 805 and officially founded the Tendai School. Jiaku and Chisho, respectively the third of its chief priests incorporated esoteric teachings into the doctrine of the Tendai School. Hence the Tendai School in Japan rapidly assumed the character of esotericism.

T'ien-t'ai

Also referred to as Chih-I, he was the founder of the T'ien-t'ai school in China. He became known for his profound lectures on the Lotus Sutra. He refuted the scriptural classifications formulated by the ten major Buddhist schools of his day and classified all of Shakyamuni Buddha's sutras into five periods and eight teachings, demonstrating the supremacy of the Lotus Sutra. His principal works, 'The Profound Meaning of The Lotus Sutra', 'The Words and Phrases of The Lotus Sutra' and 'Great Concentration and Insight', were all recorded and compiled by his immediate disciple Chang-an. In 'Great Concentration and Insight', T'ien-t'ai set forth the principle of three thousand realms in a single moment of life and the practice of meditation to realize it. It is this philosophy that is outlined in the theory of the ten worlds and the quantum mechanical scientific understanding of the Oneness of life. Both of these theories are taught on The Gateway to Enlightenment course contained within The Seekers Guide for a New Awakening. In this course we are going to focus on the concept of three thousand realms in a single moment of life to awaken the Reiki Master's wisdom.

Nam Myoho Renge Kyo is the The Lotus Sutra's Title

A Mahayana sutra that reveals the true aspect of all phenomena and Shakyamuni's true identity as the Buddha who obtained enlightenment countless eons ago, revealing the eternity of life. One of the most popular Buddhist scriptures, it maintains that all people can obtain Buddhahood. The title of the Lotus Sutra is 'Myoho Renge Kyo' meaning "The Sutra of the Lotus of the Wonderful Law".

Namu Myoho Renge Kyo

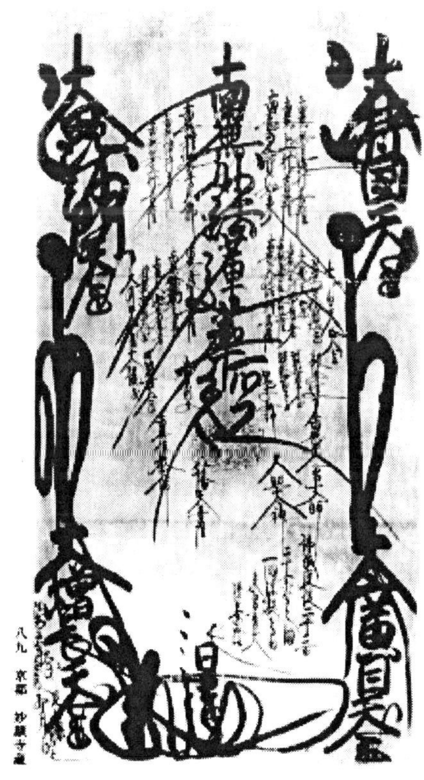

We would like to thank Nichiren Shu for permission to display the Mystic Gohonzon. Focus on this Mandala when you chant the mantra for attaining Buddhahood - **'Namu Myoho Renge Kyo'**. The pronunciation is the same as on the CD demonstration track.

The Mystic Law Mantra for Attaining Buddha Wisdom

NAMU Means devotion, to devote yourself and Myoho Renge Kyo is the title of the Lotus Sutra, which is said to contain all of the Buddhist teachings. So, in the act of chanting 'Namu Myoho Renge Kyo', we devote ourselves, fuse our lives with the fundamental law of eternity and in so doing immediately manifest our inherent Buddha nature.

MYOHO Means mystic law, to open and reveal the true entity of life, the Buddha-nature in our lives. This transforms our life condition to the Buddha state. "Myo" indicates the nature of enlightenment – Buddhahood. "Ho" indicates fundamental darkness or illusion, the first nine of the ten worlds. The Oneness of illusion and enlightenment is called MYOHO or the mystic law.

RENGE Means the workings of the Buddha state through the nine worlds in the wonderful law of creation that simultaneously, at the same time, processes both cause and effect. "Renge" embraces and illuminates the law of Karma.

KYO Means teaching, the Buddha voice, sound or vibration. Sound never stops affecting everything else in the boundless universe, through the eternal flow of life, past, present and future.

I would like to quote this profound writing that beautifully illustrates its meaning

" To practice only the seven characters of 'Namu Myoho Renge Kyo' may appear limited, yet since this law is the master of all Buddhas of the past, present and future, the teacher of all Bodhisattvas in the universe and the guide that enables all human beings to obtain Buddhahood, its practice is incomparably profound".

Welcome to the Devotional Practice of 'The Lotus Sutra'

Chanting 'Namu Myoho Renge Kyo' is the cause and enlightenment is the effect which arises instantaneously. This is because 'Namu Myoho Renge Kyo' is the law which simultaneously, at the same time, possesses both cause and effect.

This practice will develop Buddha Wisdom; it is a source of purification with the creation of joy and happiness. I would like to give you some guidelines on how to sit when you are chanting this great mystical mantra.

1. Put your hands in the prayer position in front of your heart chakra.
2. Sit with a straight back
3. You can sit in a straight back chair or on the floor, whatever you prefer
4. If you are sitting in a chair uncross your legs
5. Make sure you are comfortable as this practice is not an austerity

This practice is a celebration in the meeting and joining with Eternity – The Eternal Buddha Nature. You are reconnecting and fusing with your transcendental, essential Buddha Nature. You are now developing the Wisdom Body of the Divine Unchanging Universal Consciousness, which is the core of all creation. You are changing your destiny and transforming your soul into an enlightened being with a predominant life condition of the Buddha Nature; the soul ascends to the crown.

I promise you that with your daily practice this will happen to you within this lifetime. The real secret is simple - it is a consistent daily practice and study, no matter what, of these Universal Laws and Divine Truths contained within this course manual. It is recommended that you also study 'The Gateway to Enlightenment' and 'Love and Relationships' contained within The Seekers Guide for a New Awakening.

This practice will directly connect you to the source of creation therefore whatever you desire will quickly be realised through the Law of Attraction. The whole philosophy of Ichinen Sanzen is inscribed on the Mandala Gohonzon on page 27. Chant with your eyes open and focused upon the Mandala to awaken your deepest Buddha Wisdom. Repeatedly re-reading this manual reveals its layered meaning.

Recommended daily practice

- If you lay awake in bed in the morning and enjoy a dream-like state give yourself a Reiki healing treatment.
- When you first get up in the morning chant 'Namu Myoho Renge Kyo' for ten to fifteen minutes keeping your eyes open.

- Practice Reiki healing whenever needed throughout your day for yourself and for others, as and when required.
- Early in the evening chant 'Namu Myoho Renge Kyo' ten to fifteen minutes. During the evening when relaxing or whenever you feel the need, invoke Reiki healing.

Ichinen Sanzen - Life's Unlimited Potential

The principle of three thousand realms in a single moment of life

Quantum Physics Findings

I would like to introduce you to this beautiful theoretical concept that explains how life works and is expressed within the whole of existence. What is interesting with the new discoveries recently found in quantum physics is that we are seeing the merging of mysticism with science. From these two different approaches the concepts of life's workings agree with one another.

This is very exciting for those of us who are helping to raise the consciousness of mankind through our own personal transformation; radiating in higher consciousness. As a Reiki Master you are expanding your consciousness beyond yourself to embrace the whole world in Unconditional Love. Your power and influence will be in proportion to your inner resolve and faith. My advice is to teach as many people as you can about the mystic law of life. In a respectful manner stay away from those who dismiss you, as they will try and pull you, albeit unconsciously, into the lower life conditions of existence trying to maintain the ego's control over life.

Quantum Physics says that the whole of existence comes from the Unified Field, which is conscious. All phenomena in the cosmos come from this field and also return to it. The VIDEO movie 'What the Bleep do we know' is well worth viewing as this illustrates these new findings very well and is available on Amazon.

They have discovered that around this Unified Field, energy exists that is waving in its shape. This is similar to when a stone is thrown into a still lake - it will create ripples on the water; this waving energy is like the ripples. The still water is like the unified field or empty space. All existence consists of space, particles and waves. As waves, electrons or photons (particles of light) have no precise location, but exist as 'probability fields'. As particles, the probability field collapses into a solid object locatable in a time and space location; daily life experiences.

This discovery agrees with the Buddhist concept of the first three of the ten factors of life, as explained further on:

1. The physical = solid matter or particles
2. The nature or spiritual = the waving
3. The entity or mystic law/Divine = Unified Field or space

The other finding is that when we observe this waving field it changes shape and manifests into matter. This means that our thoughts and desires interact with this field which causes it to change, bringing into life what we had wished for. This explains the Law of Attraction. We bring into existence our own reality!

This also explains the creative relationship with the apparent separate self and the Divine. It shows us that we are really one and that if we develop Divine wisdom, suspending our ego and personal intuition, the outcomes will be influenced from our inner core of Divinity. I know what outcomes I would prefer, how about you?

This also shows us that we bring into existence our own reality, therefore we are the creative source responsible for our life; we live in our own creation. The reality we live in is state dependant. This means that the reality of our experience is determined by the world or consciousness we are resonating in. This concept is explained in the section on the Ten Worlds or Ten Life Conditions. The whole universe is actually Bliss. It is this possibility, the possibility of Unconditional Love with the manifestation of Divine Wisdom that exists for you right now.

The quantum physicists have also discovered that when our thoughts come into contact with this waving field there exist three thousand possible outcomes that could manifest, or be brought into existence, just from a single thought. A Particle, in its waving 'probability field' has been discovered to be in three thousand places at the same time. These three thousand possibilities exist at the same time in the same place. Why they do not displace each other is because they are all vibrating at a different frequency. They are the same but different.

The concept of all exclusivity and Oneness now needs to be embraced because these three thousand possible outcomes all exist at the same time and in the same place, the only difference is their vibrational frequency. This explains that it is our consciousness that determines what possibility will manifest from these three thousand possibilities of existence in a single life moment.

This explains that the opportunity for change really does exist; every outcome in your life is dependent on your consciousness, your life condition in the moment!

This concept explains 'The Power of Now' because you are experiencing your past in the present and are creating your future in the present. You are an alchemist.

The findings in The Lotus Sutra

The explanation that T'ien-t'ai taught in his 'Great Concentration and Insight' is as follows: "Life at each moment is endowed with Ten Worlds. At the same time, each of the Ten Worlds is endowed with all the others, so that an entity of life actually possesses one hundred worlds. Each of these worlds in turn possesses thirty realms of existence. These are made up of the ten factors of life and the three realms of existence; self, society and environment. The three thousand realms of existence are all possessed by a single entity of life. If there is no life, that is the end of the matter. But if there is the slightest bit of life, it contains all three thousand realms".

The Ten worlds are mutually inclusive or contained within each other. One is visible while the other nine worlds are hidden within it. This is why the possibility of one hundred worlds exists. You get the possibility of ten times ten different outcomes at any one moment of existence, this equals one hundred different possible consciousnesses or life conditions.

Ichinen Sanzen Overview

The Ten worlds are: Hell, Hunger, Animality, Egocentric Arrogance, Humanity, Heaven, Learning, Realization, Bodhisattva and Buddhahood.

The Ten Factors are: Appearance, Nature, Entity, Power, Influence, Internal Cause, Latent Effect, External Cause, Manifest Effect and Consistency from beginning to end.

The Three Realms of Existence are: Self, Society and Environment.

We are going to look into this model of existence in more detail in the following pages. You will discover that you will be able to see this model working in daily life. This will bring wisdom to the moment.

The Divine energy expresses itself as different states of awareness

The Divine Source in its essence, at its core is pure awareness but as it expresses itself into our lives, when it manifests into the world of cause and effect, duality, it expresses itself in different states of awareness. In fact the different states of awareness all exist in the same place at the same time. The only difference between them is in their consciousness function and their rate of vibration.

The Ten Worlds or life conditions – Ten states of consciousness

First of all I would like to discuss the reason why we all perceive the world in a different way from one another. This concept relates to and is very important to understanding the concept of your soul and how you perceive the world in which you live and are experiencing life.

Within the whole of existence the Buddhist highest teachings explain that existence is comprised of ten different energy vibrations or life conditions. Once again the concept of mutually inclusive is applied to these ten life conditions. The nine soul life conditions are contained within the one life condition of Buddhahood/Enlightenment, so one life condition contains all the other nine life conditions; they all occupy the same space.

What is important to understand is that at any one moment within existence any of the nine life conditions can manifest at any time and are in constant change from moment to moment within each other.

Another important concept to consider is that any of the nine worlds are contained within the realm of duality.

The tenth world in Buddhism relates to what we have been referring to as The Divine or God or The Universal Beloved Divine Consciousness.

This is very interesting because you can see that there are overlapping parallels, different names relating to the same essence. In Christianity this essence will be known as God. I deeply respect Christianity however I am unable to find an explanation of the workings of life in relation to God within their teachings. This is why I refer to Eastern philosophy and Quantum Physics.

Let us begin by explaining these ten life conditions. What is important to understand is that within every molecule of life, within every human being, within the natural environment, within the whole of creation these ten life conditions exist. So you can imagine that every interaction, every experience is being perceived according to the predominant life condition, state of awareness, which the soul is tuned into.

I would like to first of all say that through the experience of cause and effect as explained in the ten factors of life, the life condition of every action, every cause and effect experience is charged with a certain vibrational awareness or consciousness by one of the ten worlds.

This explains why different individuals display predominant perceptions relating to life. The individual soul is explained as your own personality which is a collection of all the causes and effects, known as your collective karma. Your soul is predominantly vibrating within one of the life conditions or consciousnesses that now will be explained.

As I am explaining the ten worlds meditate upon them and see if you can identify with their descriptions, their tendencies, the different ways of thinking and perceiving your life's daily experience.

Please remember that your life is not fixed in just one of these conditions because your life is constantly changing, it is in a state of constant transformation. So the world that we are experiencing now at this moment has the potential at any moment to change and manifest into one of the other nine hidden unseen life conditions.

This forms the basis for the belief that every single person has the opportunity to become a Buddha because Buddhahood exists within your own life.

All you have to do is: activate the state of Reiki healing, meditate upon wisdom philosophy, chant the mystic mantras and you will connect and activate The Beloved Divine Universal Consciousness, Spirit. This will transform the nine worlds of duality from illusion into Enlightenment.

1. Hell : Hell is a state lacking in freedom. When we are severely restricted, hell attracts a condition of extreme suffering, hopelessness, despair, frustration in which one is spurred by rage to destroy oneself or others as an attempt to break free from the feeling of being tortured. The emotional quality I would probably say is anger based upon fear. Remember fear exists in direct opposition to or the absence of love.

2. Hunger (Greed or Craving - Unsatisfied desire) : In this state of awareness we are controlled by constant cravings for objects or certain experiences; such as wealth, fame, sex, pleasure etc. Someone in this state has relentless craving and the inability to become personally satisfied even when their desire is achieved. The causes of this state of awareness are to be found in such tendencies as greed, miserliness and jealousy. Greed can lead to war and pollution within the environment.

3. Animality: In this state we are like an animal driven by survival instincts and lack any restraining virtues such as sense or reason, morality or any thought about the results of our action. People in this state only observe the law of the jungle. They have no awareness of the law of cause and effect or Karma. They are at the beck and call of those they consider superior, while they dominate those weaker than themselves.

4. Egocentric Perversion – Arrogance: In this life condition you would be dominated by a selfish ego, competitiveness, arrogance and the need to be superior in all things. In this state of awareness you are aware of the ego, but it is a distorted ego, determined to succeed over others whatever the cost. You would see everything as a potential threat to your own survival, very similar to the state of paranoia.

In this state you would only value yourself, holding everyone else in contempt, a state of self-centeredness. You would believe that you are superior to everybody else, you could not bear to be found inferior to anyone else in any respect and if you do you would look for an opportunity to challenge and destroy him or her. Revenge, domination and power are some of the negative conditions of this state of awareness. This state is a classic description of a dictator.

5. Humanity or Tranquillity: Calmness is the world of humanity. This is the life condition in which you can use reason to control your instinctive desires, so that the more truly humane qualities such as love and benevolence can emerge. People in this state of humanity exercise sound judgement, distinguish right from wrong and in general behave in a humane fashion. The negative aspect to this state is that you can become lulled into not making effort to realize your full potential. However, it is a sensitive state and you can easily fall into apathy. Furthermore, you can easily find yourself in hell if your personal life conditions are disrupted.

6. Heaven or Rapture: The pleasure you feel when your desires are fulfilled explains the experience of rapture. Think of the immense joy that you experience when, for example, you have satisfied yourself by obtaining something that you have desired for a long-time, or when long-term suffering has finally been relieved. As our desires are satisfied we become overjoyed and rapturous, yet heady and blind, failing to see the pitfalls and traps that lie ahead; we then fall back into a state of hell.

This hell state, although painful has the positive aspect of making us face reality once again. Unlike the true happiness of Buddhahood this state of heaven is only temporary and disappears with the passage of time or even the slightest change to personal circumstances.

The Six Lower Life Conditions

The first six life conditions, from hell to heaven, are called the six lower life conditions in Buddhism or six lower worlds. All of them have one thing in common: they are bought about through either fulfilling or acting out various desires and impulses. Their appearance or disappearance is therefore controlled by external circumstances.

Buddhism points out that most people spend their lives shuttling back and forth among these six lower worlds without ever realizing that they are completely at the mercy of their reactions to their environment. In effect they are purely responding to life. Any happiness or satisfaction that we may experience in these states is entirely governed by circumstances and is therefore only temporary.

So when we are trapped in the six lower life conditions we fail to realize this, instead basing our entire happiness, indeed the whole of our identity, on external factors that are by definition beyond our control. People in these conditions tend to view life as fatalistic, haphazard and have a tendency to feel powerless in respect of their own life's circumstances.

However, when you recognize that everything experienced in the six lower life conditions is impermanent, a recognition that prompts you to begin a search for lasting truth and happiness, you enter into the next two life conditions those of learning and realization.

These two life conditions along with the final two, Bodhisattva and Buddhahood are named the four noble worlds. Unlike the six lower paths or life conditions, which reflect our passive reactions to our environmental circumstances, the following four life conditions are obtained only through deliberate and continued efforts on our own behalf.

The Four Noble Worlds or Life Conditions

7. Learning: This life condition is one that requires you to dedicate yourself to create a better life to improve your self through learning from ideas, knowledge and experiences from other people and books. In this condition you would seek to learn some skill, some lasting truth or self-reformation through the teachings of others.

8. Realization: This life condition is one in which you would discover a partial truth through your own observations and efforts. You would gain wisdom through an inner knowing, the spiritual insight.

So this life condition is similar to that of learning except here we seek the truth not through other people's teachings, although they may be of assistance but through our own direct perception. The emphasis here is on our own creative nature and spiritual awakening as a result of intuitively perceiving something.

Great philosophers and scientists have often written of their sudden intuitions. Anyone can refine him or herself, develop intuitive wisdom if they make effort and discipline themselves.

The life conditions of learning and realization are closely related, but they also have a negative aspect that is whilst experiencing these states people can easily become self-centred and arrogant, thinking they have nothing else to learn. You could say that the negative side that could exist in these two life states, is that as soon as someone in learning or realization achieves what they set out to do and experiences the peaks of joy, they are vulnerable to conceit and egotism.

If our souls are strongly influenced by these two states we may find that our insight and attitude to self-improvement leads to arrogance and stubbornness. We become self-satisfied and think we know it all.

9. Bodhisattva: This life condition is characterized by a state of compassion desiring happiness for others. Conscious of the bonds that link us to everyone else, when we are in this state we realize that any happiness we enjoy on our own is illusionary and is only partial and so we divert ourselves to alleviating, removing other peoples suffering, even if it could cost us our lives. How many times have you seen the self-sacrificing martyr?

Helping others can easily lead into self-sacrifice in which a person places himself or herself unconsciously but illusionary above those who are in need, causing him or her to sink immediately into the lower states of life. So within this state you not only have the aspiration for enlightenment for yourself, but you would also devote yourself to relieving the suffering of others through compassionate, altruistic actions.

Again the negative aspects of self-sacrifice can lead to the individual disrespecting their own life and developing a condescending attitude towards others.

10. Buddhahood: When the tenth state of Buddhahood is experienced you gain the wisdom to realize the eternity of life.

This life condition has infinite compassion to direct your life towards benevolent goals, unlimited freedom throughout all of eternity, a pure state of life that nothing can corrupt and a happy and pleasant life of complete fulfilment. In this condition your life continues in perfect harmony with the rhythms of the universe and exists from the infinite past to the eternal future.

This life condition is your birthright. Buddhahood balances, integrates and transforms the workings of the previous nine worlds from a state of illusion into a condition of enlightenment.

Since no life condition is static Buddhahood cannot be thought of as a final goal but a condition that requires constant efforts on behalf of the individual.

Buddhahood Ten World's Overview

You will notice that most individuals tend to resemble the characteristics of one of the nine worlds. They tend to perceive the world from that viewpoint, they respond to the world with those tendencies. That predominant life condition resonates from the core of their soul personality because the soul is the collection of all the individuals' experiences; the sum total of their karma created from the total experiences of all their causes and effects. If for example our life tendency is to resonate in the life condition of hell, we tend to react to other people with aggression.

Buddhahood's life condition is Divine purity, indestructible happiness and the condition of perfect and absolute freedom, characterized by boundless wisdom, courage, strong life force, compassion, unconditional love and universal healing.

Because each of the ten life conditions mutually possesses the other ten, in this state even the four lower worlds will reveal their positive and fundamentally enlightened aspects.

- Hell becomes the basis for compassion
- Hunger is transformed into the desire to help others reveal their own Buddhahood
- Animality reveals instinctive wisdom

- Egocentric perversion state fuels the passion for peace and justice in society.

Everything in life, mind and body, self and the environment, living and the nonliving, cause and effect are all integrated and contained within the single life moment of the ordinary person. The first nine worlds can be considered as illusion while the tenth world of Buddhahood is enlightenment.

When we consider life with the understanding that our soul has a predominant life condition based upon one of the nine worlds that is normally in a state of illusion, the objective purpose of our life therefore is to transform our soul into the life condition of enlightenment.

Is Consciousness King? "The very earliest experience, the beginning of the universe you could say, is when pure consciousness, the unified field seeing itself, creates within its essentially unified nature the threefold structure of observer, observed and process of observation. From that, at that deepest level of reality, consciousness creates creation. There is a very intimate relationship between the observer and the observed. They are ultimately united as one inseparable wholeness at the basis of creation, which is the unified field, which is also our own innermost consciousness, the self." Dr. Hagelon

The Ten Factors of Life

The second chapter of the Lotus Sutra reveals the ten factors of life: "The true entity of all phenomena can only be understood and shared between Buddhas. This reality consists of appearance, nature, entity, power, influence, internal cause, external cause, latent effect, manifest effect and their consistency from beginning to end".

The first five factors relate to the individual self. Society too can relate to these first five factors. If you look at any organisation or group of people like a family they will also display the first five factors.

In the mantra together with the ten worlds the factors 1 to 5 are embraced by the syllables **'Myo-ho'**.

1. Appearance – Physical realm, colour form and behaviour
2. Nature – Spiritual realm, inherent disposition
3. Entity – The Buddha nature
4. Power – life's inherent capacity to take action
5. Influence – the impact upon others

The first three factors will manifest the following qualities from the life condition of Buddhahood:

1. 'Appearance' signifies the physical aspects of our lives, which is interpreted as the Buddha's enlightened property of action, emancipation, or the truth of temporary existence.
2. 'Nature' means the spiritual aspect of our lives and corresponds to the Buddha's enlightened spiritual property, wisdom or truth of non-substantiality.
3. 'Entity' refers to the entity of our lives and this corresponds to the property of the Law, the truth of the Middle Way, the Dharma nature of the Law of Enlightenment.

The workings of Cause and Effect - Karma

Factors 6 to 9 explain the workings of Karma revealing our relationship to others. They describe the workings of karma and how the actions of the self cause us to shift from one of the ten worlds to another. This is embraced as **'Renge'** in the mystic chant.

6. Internal Cause – (contains latent effect at the same time)
7. Relation or External Cause (the potential for change)
8. Latent Effect
9. Manifest Effect – Becomes the internal cause with its latent effect

We have already discussed that we create our own reality and therefore the world is the result of our collective creation. This can also be known as our collective Karma; the manifest effect of all our causes and effects.

We have looked at the importance of our consciousness in the creation of our existence in the ten worlds. You will now see the relationship with the ten worlds and the law of cause and effect. The outcome of the planet is dependent upon the collective life condition of everyone on the earth. All social systems, villages, towns, cities and countries will reflect their predominant world or life condition. They will all manifest the fist five factors and interact with others individually or collectively through the law of karma, factors six to nine.

One important consideration to learn is that cause and effect exists at the same time! To many the mind is unable to understand this concept because it measures everything in a linear way, through division and separation. You did this to me and as a result I had this experience.

In reality no duality exists. The internal cause contains the latent effect. They are vibrating and manifest into existence like a seed flowering when the external relationship is right to enable it to grow. The four factors of cause and effect, the workings of karma, can be considered as follows:

- The sum total of our life's experiences is contained within our soul.
- Every life moment has been experienced from a certain consciousness, one of the ten worlds.
- Each past experience therefore has been charged with a certain vibrational frequency.
- The past experience came into existence as the result of a relationship, an external cause.
- The external cause or relationship was attracted by the internal cause.
- The result of the internal cause and the external cause coming together created the outcome or manifest effect.
- The manifest effect was already dormant within the soul as the latent effect.
- The opportunity for change is therefore consciousness dependant; this proves life is not fated.
- Fate is the result of no change in consciousness and explains repeated negative patterns of behaviour due to residing in the lower worlds and only reacting to the external cause, the external relationship of life.

- The mystical reality of enlightenment is based upon the inner change. When you change on the inside the outside naturally changes. This means everything is dependent upon your life condition. Raise your life condition to a higher consciousness and you change the latent cause and latent effect within your soul before it has come into contact with the external cause. The manifest effect eventually then becomes enlightenment.

The Oneness of Life

The above nine factors are equally endowed within all things. This is the final factor representing the totality of all the others.

In the mantra this factor is chanted as **'Kyo'.**

10. Their consistency from beginning to end – all factors exist as wholeness.

This can be seen as the Oneness of the three aspects of: spiritual nature, material appearance and entity. This factor is the integrating factor that unites the other nine in every moment of life. In other words, where there is one factor all other factors must exist.

As we have said, the first three factors, appearance, nature and entity, together make up what life is. However, these three factors are not on the same plane. Appearance (life's physical aspect) and nature (life's spiritual aspect) cannot simply be combined to form entity: entity (the changeless reality or ultimate truth of life) actually gives rise to the phenomena of appearance and nature – that is, they are its manifestations.

Power, influence, internal cause, relation, latent effect and manifest effect all represent the functions of life, but these, too, exist on different planes from each other. For example power is latent in life whereas influence is power's manifestation directed towards our surroundings. Similarly, (internal cause) and (latent effect) are both unseen in life, while (manifest effect) is the outcome we can see as a result of our seen relationship (external cause).

T'ien-tai's Profound Meaning of the Lotus Sutra wrote: "Appearance exists only in what is material; nature exists only in what is spiritual. Entity, power, influence and relation in principle combine both material and the spiritual. Internal cause and latent effect are purely spiritual; manifest effect exists in what is material".

Finally the last factor, 'consistency from beginning to end', in integrating all the others, demonstrates that both beginning and end are inseparable, revealing Oneness. The first three factors combine as entity, or beginning. The following six factors act as the functions of all phenomena, or end.

There are three different ways to look at anything therefore; peace and happiness never come from insisting only on equality or from only insisting on difference.

1. Equality: Everyone possesses the Buddha nature therefore are equal
2. Difference: Personal experience, soul disposition, the Karmic difference
3. The Totality: All things are equal but different – inclusive

We have to realise this equality within the differences and the differences within equality. Knowing individual differences but respecting his or her interests, talents, education and physical condition is the way forward in the creation of peace and harmony; to respect other peoples' different cultures, backgrounds and languages.

Key Points for Meditation

- Everything is constantly changing
- All things exist because of relationships with and to others
- The Buddha nature – the unchanging reality within all things from moment to moment

The Three Realms of Existence

1. SELF: The realm of the five components
2. SOCIETY: The realm of all living beings (sentient beings)
3. NATURE: The realm of the environment (non-sentient life)

The Self contains five components:

1. Form – life's physical aspect – four elements
2. Perception – receiving information through the sense organs
3. Conception – Creation of ideas – concepts
4. Volition – how we act and our response
5. Consciousness is the function of discernment; understanding is reflected by the ten worlds. It integrates Perception Conception and Volition.

The Self in separation

Our consciousness of the 'Self' forms the framework whereby we support our dualistic world-view of life. Our perceived division of the Universe into two parts 'self' and 'others', or internal and external arises from our consciousness of 'self'. This consciousness also gives rise to other dualities: for example, the duality of the mind and the body (in which we regard our mind as being our true self whereas the body is not), the duality of the material and the spiritual, or duality of mankind and nature. Newtonian physics, dualistic and separate thinking, is what our modern civilization is based upon, it is also the root of many present crises.

The concept of Ichinen Sanzen and modern quantum physics points the way to the resolution of such crises that exist today by demonstrating the truth that our lives are not limited to the self alone but encompass other people, the world and the Universe; the concept of Oneness.

Nichiren Daishonin writes: "Life at each moment encompasses both body and spirit and both self and the environment of all sentient beings in every condition of life, as well as non-sentient beings – plants, sky, stars and earth, on down to the most minute particles of dust. Life at each moment permeates the Universe and is revealed in all phenomena."

His point is that the individual's life at each moment simultaneously both permeates the entire Universe and encompasses within itself all the laws and phenomena of the Universe. It is, therefore, literally coextensive with the Universe. This relationship between the microcosm of human life and the macrocosm of the Universe is mystical.

The Self has nine consciousnesses, nine levels of discernment:

- The first five consciousnesses correspond to the five senses of sight, hearing, smell, taste and touch.
- The sixth consciousness integrates the perceptions of the five senses into coherent images and makes judgements about the external world.
- The seventh consciousness corresponds to the inner spiritual world and generates awareness of the self and the ability to distinguish positive from negative.
- The eighth consciousness, called alaya-consciousness, receives the results of one's positive and negative deeds and stores them as karmic potentials or 'seeds', which then produce the rewards of either happiness or suffering accordingly.
- The ninth consciousness, called amala-consciousness, which remains free from all karmic impurity, is defined as the basis of all life's functions and is identified with the true aspect of life, or the Buddha nature.

The Oneness of self and society

The reality is that we need others to live is a truth. The reality that we all experience life as individuals is easily understood, however the true reality is that we are one-being in relationship with each other; one family on earth. What we do to others is reflected back to us through the law of cause and effect. When we deliberately hurt another we only hurt ourselves.

As the ten factors reveal we require relationships to manifest our life's experiences. Without others we would not be able to experience the ten worlds. Most importantly it is other people who enable us to reveal our true identity beyond our apparent separation; that of the Divine.

The Oneness of life and the environment

It is a common human failing to always blame our sufferings on things outside ourselves, other people, or circumstances beyond our control, rather than to make the effort to look for the causes within ourselves. However, if we take the Oneness of life as a principle and base our lives on this perception, we see that the fundamental cause of all our trials and tribulations lies in ourselves and not the environment.

This principle of Oneness explains how individuals can positively influence their environments through inner change or through changing their basic life condition. This is because the individual has the potential to live in any of the ten worlds; when an individual changes in consciousness this is then reflected within the environment. Once understood this concept becomes very empowering in terms of your ability to bring about change and create value in life and the natural environment.

Nichiren Daishonin writes: "If the minds of the people are impure, their land is also impure, but if their minds are pure, so is their land. There are not two lands, pure and impure in themselves. The difference lies solely in the positive or negative of our minds."

"All non sentient phenomena are environment and the sentient beings are life. Environment is like the shadow and life the body. Without the body there can be no shadow. Similarly, without life, environment cannot exist, even though life is supported by its environment."

How life works through and from the ten life conditions

Buddhism states that there is a connection between the mind and body of each person; that a spiritual connection exists between every person in the world and that spiritual connection exists between yourself, society and the natural world that is your environment.

We tend to think that our skin is the boundary between our lives and the lives of others, in fact it is not! From a spiritual aspect when we look at nature; at that very moment nature becomes part of our lives and we are part of nature. This is because the ten worlds exist within nature as well as our lives.

Because of this relationship our lives and the environment become like a body and its shadow; the environment being passive only reacts to our life condition. The environment becomes like a mirror to ourselves. We draw out like magnetism the life condition that we are living in. How many times have you walked into a room and felt a depressed state of vibration, the whole room feels depressed because the person who was living there vibrates in their life condition of depression.

Nothing exists in isolation. Each individual person functions to bring into being the environment that in turn sustains all of the existences. All things are mutually supportive and related forming a living cosmos.

The individual life of every person contains the memory of their eternal past, storing many lifetimes of experience and different beliefs within their spiritual body. These are stored like seeds containing information of experience waiting to grow in the physical world within society.

This explains the individual differences of each person; it explains our individual character, physical appearance, our different beliefs, our likes and dislikes and why our parents are our parents.

It is the life condition and the behavioural tendency of our past experiences, which link together and grow in daily life when triggered by the same or opposite tendency within other people. The natural environment, places, can also have this effect as they too have a memory.

We need relationships to exist and become happy

In other words we all need others to live out our lives. We need relationships to exist and become happy. In the West we have the tendency to blame unpleasant experiences on our relationships with others, for example, he or she did this or that, but in reality the truth is that the spiritual seeds within our own individual lives have come to the surface in this physical world. Those spiritual seeds contain at the same time cause and effect, being charged with an emotional life condition from one of the ten worlds.

Looking at your daily life in this way you can come to understand that in reality whatever happens to you is as a result of what already exists within your own soul body because you have created it in your past.

Modern scientific thinking is able to explain the cause affecting life's workings, how something has happened. Buddhism goes one stage further in explaining why events happen. To illustrate, let's assume that an accident or disaster has occurred. A logical scientific theory of causation can be used to pursue and identify how the accident occurred, but is silent regarding why certain individuals find themselves caught up in the tragic event. Buddhism answers this question.

Buddhism teaches that it is the life condition of our heart and mind that determines our happiness. It is also true that this condition of heart and mind is what determines the quality of the natural world that exists to support human life in terms of food, medicine and nourishment. Each moment of life becomes very precious to a Buddhist because they understand that it contains the eternity of life.

Viewing life in this way illustrates that the past and the future are contained within the present moment. It could be said that our children are messages from the future.

Every event, every moment of experience becomes a spiritual seed that is contained in storage within our soul. When the seeds are in storage they are invisible but still exist, only waiting for the external relationship to vibrate them back into the physical world. This is where the idea of a circle of events is derived from.

The key point to remember is that you have the opportunity in the moment for transformation and change. The change ultimately that you will seek will be in relation to the life condition of that spiritual seed of karma from one of illusion to that of enlightenment, Buddhahood.

So Buddhism teaches you that you have a choice - everything is up to you. It becomes a life of personal responsibility because you have the power within you to change your life and create it from moment to moment how you want it to be.

Initially this could be difficult and require a lot of effort because you are attempting to transform the predominant life condition of your soul into the life condition of a Buddha. I expect you now realize that with each positive transformation of each individual spiritual seed your soul will become lighter.

Buddhism teaches that you can become reactive or passive to life becoming trapped by your environment within the six lower worlds, or you can make effort and create your life with the freedom of your Buddha nature and fly into the sky of enlightenment, absolute happiness.

We all influence and affect each other in this world, therefore making a positive change to your own life will vibrate throughout the whole universe and this contains the concept of world peace. World peace is achieved within yourself. From the point of enlightenment your influence and effect upon others will be astounding.

Spiritual Practices to
Transform Your Soul's Predominant Life Condition

Practice Balancing your Emotional Body Heart Chakra using Dai-Ko-Myo

Practice Chanting 'Namu Myoho Renge Kyo' To Open Buddha Wisdom

Reiki Master Teacher Preparation

Preparation before giving the Reiki Attunements

How to prepare the room you use for the initiations

Create an altar: Prepare an area and cover it with an altar cloth; you could use a picture of Dr Usui, some candles to represent universal wisdom, water to represent the purification of our being, you could offer incense to represent compassion. (Be careful not to overpower the area with strong fragrance that could cause discomfort to the receiver at the attunement. Incense is best offered before the attunement when you are empowering the room with your symbols). Finally you could offer real flowers for beauty and harmony; flowers also represent the ever changing nature of life.

(Don't forget to Reiki everything)

Creating a sacred space when a separate room is used for attunements. This example prepares the room with the chairs facing the altar:

1. First prepare yourself with Reiki and prayer by asking for the Reiki Guides to assist you in creating a sacred space.
2. Create a circle that includes your altar area.
3. Facing the altar open the area with a large Cho-Ku-Rei, then draw Dai-Ko-Myo.
4. Still facing the altar you walk backwards until you are standing behind the chairs that the students will sit on when they have their attunement. You then draw Sei-He-Kei and Hon-Sha-Ze-Sho-Nen.
5. Still facing the altar you walk back another two steps to the edge of your circle and draw another Hon-Sha-Ze-Sho-Nen symbol finishing off with a large Cho-Ku-Rei. Then beam energy into the circle.
6. To finish, walk around the circle to seal in the energy and intend its sacredness.

Creating a sacred space if the same room is used for attunements as well as for the group workshop work

1. First prepare yourself with Reiki and prayer by asking for the Reiki Guides to assist you in creating a sacred space.
2. Open the central area with a large Cho-Ku-Rei, then draw Dai-Ko-Myo.
3. Open any wall with a large Cho-Ku-Rei, then draw Dai-Ko-Myo. Repeat this for each wall, floor and the ceiling. (Chant the mantra to space clear the area)
4. With your chairs arranged in a circle stand behind each chair in turn and draw Sei-He-Kei and Hon-Sha-Ze-Sho-Nen.
5. Walk to the edge of the room and draw another Hon-Sha-Ze-Sho-Nen symbol finishing off with a large Cho-Ku-Rei. Then beam energy into the circle.
6. To finish, walk around the circle to seal in the energy and intend its sacredness.

Notes on using a single space for attunements and energy work

Arrange your chairs in a circle for the introductions so that everyone is facing each other. Using the same chairs it is best to arrange them before the attunement so that the person is facing towards the wall with their backs to the centre of the circle. In other words just turn them round making sure you have enough space to walk around all sides the chair.

You could ask the group to leave the room just before the attunement so you can create a sacred space for their Reiki attunement. Stand behind each chair in turn and draw Sei-Hei-Ki and Hon-Sha-Ze-Sho-Nen. Doing this will build expectation and wonder in the group and can empower the attunement experience. Only do this if there is an appropriate area the group can wait in without too much discomfort.

Invoking and intending the Reiki symbols from the Divine Chakra

In step 2 of all the attunements you start by drawing the three symbols in the air high over the crown chakra. Above the crown chakra exists a Divine chakra that connects the individual to the unchanging source of Unconditional Love. Within this realm exists the purity of Divine beings, Ascendant Masters, Reiki Guides and Angelic Beings. When you draw the Reiki symbols into this chakra you will invoke the assistance of Divine beings to assist you in the attunement.

Each symbol has a different Divine vibration so when you draw the Reiki symbols you are in fact calling that aspect of the Divine to manifest for you within the Divine chakra. Through doing this the energy vibration of each symbol will then be present and will be channelled to each chakra within the attunement initiation process.

Please consider this step of the attunement preparation as sacred as you are calling upon the realm of Divinity when you do this. The purity of your intention in this step of the attunement will definitely affect the quality of the attunement you are about to channel.

How to prepare for the initiations and attunements

1. Step in front of the altar and then prepare yourself with Reiki and prayer asking for the Reiki Guides to assist you in this attunement.
2. Remind people to put their feet on the floor with their legs uncrossed and close their eyes.
3. You can start the attunement with your own prayer out loud: - example "Let the Universal Light and Love be with us now" or "Reiki Guides assist me in this attunement".
4. The following 3 Symbols are referred to in this manual as (4, 3 & 1) which are Dai-Ko-Myo, Hon-Sha-Ze-Sho-Nen & Cho-Ku-Rei. Use them in this order for all attunements.
5. In step 2 of all the attunements you draw these three symbols high in the air over the crown before you start the attunement; this intention acts as if they are in a holding reservoir waiting for you to channel them down at each step of the attunement.
6. Visualize or imagine the symbols in Golden light and chant their mantra silently three times as you channel each symbol at each step of the attunement.
7. Before each stage of the attunement chant the mantra Cho-Ku-Rei three times as you draw its symbol over the chakra that is to be attuned. This opens the chakra to receive the 3 symbols energy (4, 3 & 1) being channelled.

Notes for Your Interest

Reiki First Degree given as one or three attunements

The traditional method of transferring the Reiki First Degree attunement is completed over two days in three parts, (known as three/four attunements). We teach the complete traditional approach but also endorse the single attunement as complete in itself which is acceptable for professional certification.

It is the third of the First Degree Reiki attunements that is complete in itself and can be given on its own. This attunement opens the crown, the throat, the third eye, the heart and the hand chakras. You will find a full explanation of how to transfer this single attunement on page 53 entitled 'Reiki 1st Degree – All the ten steps for one attunement'.

Reiki First Degree attunements that are given as three attunements over two days are better for the client as it allows time for their energy field to adjust and deepen to the Reiki energy.

When giving three attunements over two days:

1. The first attunement is given on the first day in the morning; this opens the crown, the heart and the hands chakras.
2. The second attunement is given on day one in the afternoon; this opens the crown, the throat, the heart and the hands chakras.
3. The third attunement is given on day two in the morning and this opens all the chakras; the crown, the throat, the third eye, the heart and the hands.

You will see that the throat chakra is added in the second attunement and the third eye chakra is added in the third attunement.

The Chakra Retains a Reiki Energy Memory Connection

Just as your mind and the cells in your body have a memory, the energy centres, the chakras also have a memory. What is happening in an attunement is that you are attuning the chakra to recognise the energy vibration of the Reiki energy. Once recognised or attuned the Chakra has a memory connection for life. The client can then turn on their Reiki energy by their intention to do so at any time, because the memory connection is retained within their chakras.

How to Transfer the Attunements

Reiki 1st Degree - All the Ten Steps for One Attunement

Step 1 - Opening the Aura
Draw a Large Cho-Ku-Rei over the Heart Chakra and Body

1. Ask the receiver to close their eyes before you start and then smooth down their aura.
2. Draw a large Cho-Ku-Rei over the heart chakra at the front of body to open the aura.
3. Beam Reiki healing energy to the heart area and front of body; this helps to open the heart chakra and the whole aura.

Step 2 – Right or Left Hand on Right or Left Shoulder - Other Hand Draws 3 Symbols in the air invoking Divine Chakra channelling.

Walk (to your right) anticlockwise round client and place your right or left hand on their right or left shoulder and as you do this draw the 3 symbols in the air chanting their mantras 3 times using your left or right hand in the following order; Dai-Ko-Myo, Hon-Sha-Ze-Sho-Nen & Cho-Ku-Rei.

Step 3 - Opening the Crown Chakra

1. Draw a small Cho-Ku-Rei over the crown to open the chakra
2. Cup your hands over the crown and channel the 3 symbols (4, 3 & 1) down through the whole body. (Visualize the symbols in Golden light and chant their mantra three times silently as you channel each symbol into the crown.)

Step 4 - Both hands on shoulders to prepare opening the heart Chakra

1. Place both hands on shoulders, fingers on collar bone to send energy to heart.

2. Channel the 3 symbols (4, 3 & 1) down the body into the heart. This helps open and attune the lower chakras.

Step 5 - Opening the Throat Chakra

1. Walk (to your right) anticlockwise to side of their body stopping in line with their shoulders and open throat with Cho-Ku-Rei. Place one hand in front and one hand at back of their throat (both hands approx. 3" - 10 cm off the body)
2. Channel the 3 symbols (4, 3 & 1)

Step 6 - Opening The Third Eye Chakra

1. Draw Cho-Ku-Rei to open third eye and then place one hand on Third eye and one hand at back of head cupping just up from the base (Near T1 Medulla Oblongata)
2. Channel the 3 symbols (4, 3 & 1) - Into third eye - Inside head between your two hands

Step 7 - Opening The Heart Chakra

1. Move to front of body. Draw Cho-Ku-Rei to open chakra
2. Hold both hands 3" (10 cm) over heart chakra & Channel the 3 symbols (4, 3 & 1)

Step 8 - Opening The Hand Chakras

1. Put client's hands in prayer position and Draw Cho-Ku-Rei over them
2. Hand position 1 (see VIDEO) Your right hand – place your fingers on the tips of their fingers; your little finger is sitting on their index finger. Your left hand – Place your thumb across the top of their thumbs and wrap your hand around their hands. Channel the 3 symbols (4, 3 & 1)
3. Hand position 2 (see VIDEO) Lay your left hand thumb across the tips of their fingers – the tip of your thumb will be placed on their first finger so that you can then wrap your hand around theirs. Your right hand ring and middle finger tips are placed on their thumbs. Channel the 3 symbols (4, 3 & 1)

Step 9 - Blowing the Breath of Life and Filling the Aura

1. Draw a large Cho-Ku-Rei over solar plexus and sacral chakra (belly). Beam energy to that chakra holding the energy in that place with your hands.
2. Draw a Cho-Ku-Rei with the tip of your tongue at the top of your upper teeth on the roof of your mouth and then blow it into the solar plexus and up the body. This step b) is optional.
3. Wrap both your hands gently around their hands and blow a Cho-Ku-Rei into their Heart chakra across the tips of their fingers. Move their hands up so that the tips of their fingers are in line with their third eye and blow a Cho-Ku-Rei into the third eye. Move their hands up so that the tips of their fingers are in line with their crown and blow a Cho-Ku-Rei into the crown. Put their hands back down in original prayer position in front of their heart chakra to finish.

Step 10 - Grounding the client

Draw a large Cho-Ku-Rei over aura in front of the heart to ground them. Indicate that the hands can come down in their laps and they can open their eyes in their own time.

Optional Finish after attunement

Test for Reiki 1st and 2nd degree, this allows the client to feel their Reiki energy as demonstrated on the tutorial VIDEO.

1. After the client is fully present ask them to hold their hands vertically, palms facing each other about 6" apart with their fingers pointing at you. Both hands are about level with the solar plexus or whatever is comfortable for them. You are going to test their sensitivity by bringing your hand slowly between theirs starting from about two feet away from their hands. Ask them now to close their eyes and tell you when they can feel your energy as your hand moves closer between theirs. When the client says "Now" keep your hand still. Ask them to open their eyes so they can see how close your hand is to their energy field. Then you can play in-between their hands in their energy field and ask them how it feels.

2. Now ask them to close their eyes again and to switch their Reiki on and put their hands over their eyes until they can feel the Reiki energy. When they have done this ask them "How did it feel to you?"

Reiki 1st Degree – 3 Separate Attunements Over Two Days

First Attunement - Day One AM

Step 1 - Opening the Aura
Large Cho-Ku-Rei over the Heart Chakra and Body

1. Ask the receiver to close their eyes before you start and then smooth down their aura.
2. Draw a large Cho-Ku-Rei over the heart chakra at the front of body to open the aura.
3. Beam Reiki healing energy to the heart area and front of body; this helps to open the heart chakra and the whole aura.

Step 2 – Right or Left Hand on Right or Left Shoulder - Other Hand Draws 3 Symbols in the air invoking Divine Chakra channelling

Walk (to your right) anticlockwise round client and place your right or left hand on their right or left shoulder and as you do this draw the 3 symbols in the air chanting their mantras 3 times using your left or right hand in the following order; Dai-Ko-Myo, Hon-Sha-Ze-Sho-Nen and Cho-Ku-Rei.

Step 3 - Opening the Crown Chakra

1. Draw a small Cho-Ku-Rei over the crown to open the chakra
2. Cup your hands over the crown and channel the 3 symbols (4, 3 & 1) down through the whole body. (Visualize the symbols in Golden light and chant their mantra three times silently as you channel each symbol into the crown.)

Step 4 - Both hands on shoulders to prepare opening the heart Chakra

1. Place both hands on shoulders, fingers on collar bone to send energy to heart.
2. Channel the 3 symbols (4, 3 & 1) down the body into the heart. This helps open and attune the lower chakras.

Step 7 - Opening The Heart Chakra

1. Move to front of body. Draw Cho-Ku-Rei to open chakra.
2. Hold both hands 3" (10 cm) over heart chakra and Channel the 3 symbols (4, 3 & 1)

Step 8 - Opening The Hand Chakras

1. Put client's hands in prayer position and Draw Cho-Ku-Rei over them
2. Hand position 1 (see VIDEO) Your right hand – place your fingers on the tips of their fingers; your little finger is sitting on their index finger. Your left hand – Place your thumb across the top of their thumbs and wrap your hand around their hands. Channel the 3 symbols (4, 3 & 1)
3. Hand position 2 (see VIDEO) Lay your left hand thumb across the tips of their fingers – the tip of your thumb will be placed on their first finger so that you can then wrap your hand around theirs. Your right hand ring and middle finger tips are placed on their thumbs. Channel the 3 symbols (4, 3 & 1)

Step 9 - Blowing the Breath of Life & Filling the Aura

1. Draw a large Cho-Ku-Rei over solar plexus and sacral chakra (belly). Beam energy to that chakra holding the energy in that place with your hands.
2. Draw a Cho-Ku-Rei with the tip of your tongue at the top of your upper teeth on the roof of your mouth and then blow it into the solar plexus and up the body. This step b) is optional.
3. Wrap both your hands gently around their hands and blow a Cho-Ku-Rei into their Heart chakra across the tips of their fingers. Move their hands up so that the tips of their fingers are in line with their third eye and blow a Cho-Ku-Rei into the third eye. Move their hands up so that the tips of their fingers are in line with their crown and blow a Cho-Ku-Rei into the crown. Put their hands back down in original prayer position in front of their heart chakra to finish.

Step 10 - Grounding the client

Draw a large Cho-Ku-Rei over aura in front of the heart to ground them. Indicate that the hands can come down in their laps and they can open their eyes in their own time.

Reiki 1st Degree Second Attunement - Day One PM

Step 1 - Opening the Aura
Draw a Large Cho-Ku-Rei over the Heart Chakra and Body

1. Ask the receiver to close their eyes before you start and then smooth down their aura.
2. Draw a large Cho-Ku-Rei over the heart chakra at the front of body to open the aura.
3. Beam Reiki healing energy to the heart area and front of body; this helps to open the heart chakra and the whole aura.

Step 2 – Right or Left Hand on Right or Left Shoulder - Other Hand Draws 3 Symbols in the air invoking Divine Chakra channelling

Walk (to your right) anticlockwise round client and place your right or left hand on their right or left shoulder and as you do this draw the 3 symbols in the air chanting their mantras 3 times using your left or right hand in the following order, Dai-Ko-Myo, Hon-Sha-Ze-Sho-Nen and Cho-Ku-Rei.

Step 3 - Opening the Crown Chakra

1. Draw a small Cho-Ku-Rei over the crown to open the chakra
2. Cup your hands over the crown and channel the 3 symbols (4, 3 & 1) down through the whole body. (Visualize the symbols in Golden light and chant their mantra three times silently as you channel each symbol into the crown.)

Step 4 Both hands on shoulders to prepare opening the heart Chakra

1. Place both hands on shoulders, fingers on collar bone to send energy to heart.
2. Channel the 3 symbols (4, 3 & 1) down the body into the heart. This helps open and attune the lower chakras.

Step 5 - Opening the Throat Chakra

1. Walk (to your right) anticlockwise to side of their body stopping in line with their shoulders and open throat with Cho-Ku-Rei. Place one hand in front and one hand at back of their throat (both hands approx. 3" - 10 cm off the body)
2. Channel the 3 symbols (4, 3 & 1)

Step 7 - Opening The Heart Chakra

1. Move to front of body. Draw Cho-Ku-Rei to open chakra
2. Hold both hands 3" (10 cm) over heart chakra & Channel the 3 symbols (4, 3 & 1)

Step 8 - Opening The Hand Chakras

1. Put client's hands in prayer position and Draw Cho-Ku-Rei over them
2. Hand position 1 (see VIDEO) Your right hand – place your fingers on the tips of their fingers; your little finger is sitting on their index finger. Your left hand – Place your thumb across the top of their thumbs and wrap your hand around their hands. Channel the 3 symbols (4, 3 & 1)
3. Hand position 2 (see VIDEO) Lay your left hand thumb across the tips of their fingers – the tip of your thumb will be placed on their first finger so that you can then wrap your hand around theirs. Your right hand ring and middle finger tips are placed on their thumbs. Channel the 3 symbols (4, 3 & 1)

Step 9 - Blowing the Breath of Life and Filling the Aura

1. Draw a large Cho-Ku-Rei over solar plexus and sacral chakra (belly). Beam energy to that chakra holding the energy in that place with your hands.
2. Draw a Cho-Ku-Rei with the tip of your tongue at the top of your upper teeth on the roof of your mouth and then blow it into the solar plexus and up the body. This step b) is optional.
3. Wrap both your hands gently around their hands and blow a Cho-Ku-Rei into their Heart chakra across the tips of their fingers. Move their hands up so that the tips of their fingers are in line with their third eye and blow a Cho-Ku-Rei into the third eye. Move their hands up so that the tips of their fingers are in line with their crown and blow a Cho-Ku-Rei into the crown. Put their hands back down in original prayer position in front of their heart chakra to finish.

Step 10 - Grounding the client

Draw a large Cho-Ku-Rei over aura in front of the heart to ground them. Indicate that the hands can come down in their laps and they can open their eyes in their own time.

Reiki 1st Degree Third Attunement Day Two AM

Step 1 - Opening the Aura

Draw a Large Cho-Ku-Rei over the Heart Chakra and Body

1. Ask the receiver to close their eyes before you start and then smooth down their aura.
2. Draw a large Cho-Ku-Rei over the heart chakra at the front of body to open the aura.
3. Beam Reiki healing energy to the heart area and front of body; this helps to open the heart chakra and the whole aura.

Step 2 – Right or Left Hand on Right or Left Shoulder - Other Hand Draws 3 Symbols in the air invoking Divine Chakra channelling

Walk (to your right) anticlockwise round client and place your right or left hand on their right or left shoulder and as you do this draw the 3 symbols in the air chanting their mantras 3 times using your left or right hand in the following order; Dai-Ko-Myo, Hon-Sha-Ze-Sho-Nen and Cho-Ku-Rei.

Step 3 - Opening the Crown Chakra

1. Draw a small Cho-Ku-Rei over the crown to open the chakra
2. Cup your hands over the crown and channel the 3 symbols (4, 3 & 1) down through the whole body. (Visualize the symbols in Golden light and chant their mantra three times silently as you channel each symbol into the crown.)

Step 4 Both hands on shoulders to prepare opening the heart Chakra

1. Place both hands on shoulders, fingers on collar bone to send energy to heart.
2. Channel the 3 symbols (4, 3 & 1) down the body into the heart. This helps open and attune the lower chakras.

Step 5 - Opening the Throat Chakra

1. Walk (to your right) anticlockwise to side of their body stopping in line with their shoulders and open throat with Cho-Ku-Rei. Place one hand in front and one hand at back of their throat (both hands approx. 3" 10 cm off the body)
2. Channel the 3 symbols (4, 3 & 1)

Step 6 - Opening The Third Eye Chakra

1. Draw Cho-Ku-Rei to open third eye & then place one hand on third eye and one hand at back of head cupping just up from the base (Near T1 Medulla Oblongata)
2. Channel the 3 symbols (4, 3 & 1) - Into third eye - Inside head between your two hands

Step 7 - Opening The Heart Chakra

1. Move to front of body. Draw Cho-Ku-Rei to open chakra
2. Hold both hands 3" (10 cm) over heart chakra and Channel the 3 symbols (4, 3 & 1)

Step 8 - Opening The Hand Chakras

1. Put client's hands in prayer position and Draw Cho-Ku-Rei over them
2. Hand position 1 (see VIDEO) Your right hand – place your fingers on the tips of their fingers; your little finger is sitting on their index finger. Your left hand – Place your thumb across the top of their thumbs and wrap your hand around their hands. Channel the 3 symbols (4, 3 & 1)
3. Hand position 2 (see VIDEO) Lay your left hand thumb across the tips of their fingers – the tip of your thumb will be placed on their first finger so that you can then wrap your hand around theirs. Your right hand ring and middle finger tips are placed on their thumbs. Channel the 3 symbols (4, 3 & 1)

Step 9 - Blowing the Breath of Life & Filling the Aura

1. Draw a large Cho-Ku-Rei over solar plexus and sacral chakra (belly). Beam energy to that chakra holding the energy in that place with your hands.
2. Draw a Cho-Ku-Rei with the tip of your tongue at the top of your upper teeth on the roof of your mouth and then blow it into the solar plexus and up the body. This step b) is optional.
3. Wrap both your hands gently around their hands and blow a Cho-Ku-Rei into their Heart chakra across the tips of their fingers. Move their hands up so that the tips of their fingers are in line with their third eye and blow a Cho-Ku-Rei into the third eye. Move their hands up so that the tips of their fingers are in line with their crown and blow a Cho-Ku-Rei into the crown. Put their hands back down in original prayer position in front of their heart chakra to finish.

Step 10 - Grounding the Client

Draw a large Cho-Ku-Rei over aura in front of the heart to ground them. Indicate that the hands can come down in their laps and they can open their eyes in their own time.

Optional Finish After the Attunement

Test for Reiki 1st and 2nd degree, this allows the client to feel their Reiki energy as demonstrated on the tutorial Video.

1. After the client is fully present ask them to hold their hands vertically, palms facing each other about 6" apart with their fingers pointing at you. Both hands are about level with the solar plexus or whatever is comfortable for them. You are going to test their sensitivity by bringing your hand slowly between theirs starting from about two feet away from their hands. Ask them now to close their eyes and tell you when they can feel your energy as your hand moves closer between theirs. When the client says "Now" keep your hand still. Ask them to open their eyes so they can see how close your hand is to their energy field. Then you can play in-between their hands in their energy field and ask them how it feels.

2. Now ask them to close their eyes again and to switch their Reiki on and put their hands over their eyes until they can feel the Reiki energy. When they have done this ask them "How did it feel to you?"

Reiki 2nd Degree Attunement

Step 1 - Opening the Aura

Draw a Large Cho-Ku-Rei over the Heart Chakra and Body

1. Ask the receiver to close their eyes before you start and then smooth down their aura.
2. Draw a large Cho-Ku-Rei over the heart chakra at the front of body to open the aura.
3. Beam Reiki healing energy to the heart area and front of body; this helps to open the heart chakra and the whole aura.

Step 2 – Right or Left Hand on Right or Left Shoulder - Other Hand Draws 3 Symbols in the air invoking Divine Chakra channelling

Walk (to your right) anticlockwise round client and place your right or left hand on their right or left shoulder and as you do this draw the 3 symbols in the air chanting their mantras 3 times using your left or right hand in the following order; Dai-Ko-Myo, Hon-Sha-Ze-Sho-Nen & Cho-Ku-Rei.

Step 3 - Opening the Crown Chakra

1. Draw a small Cho-Ku-Rei over the crown to open the chakra
2. Cup your hands over the crown and channel the 3 symbols (4, 3 & 1) down through the whole body. (Visualize the symbols in Golden light and chant their mantra three times silently as you channel each symbol into the crown.)

Step 4 - Both hands on shoulders to prepare opening the heart Chakra

1. Place both hands on shoulders, fingers on collar bone to send energy to heart.
2. Channel the 3 symbols (4, 3 & 1) down the body into the heart. This helps open and attune the lower chakras.

Step 5 - Opening the Throat Chakra

1. Walk (to your right) anticlockwise to side of their body stopping in line with their shoulders and open throat with Cho-Ku-Rei. Place one hand in front and one hand at back of their throat (both hands approx. 3" - 10 cm off the body)
2. Channel the 3 symbols (4, 3 & 1)

Step 6 - Opening The Third Eye Chakra

1. Draw Cho-Ku-Rei to open third eye & then place one hand on Third eye and one hand at back of head cupping just up from the base (Near T1 Medulla Oblongata)
2. Channel the 3 symbols (4, 3 & 1) - Into third eye - Inside head between your two hands

Step 7 - Opening The Heart Chakra

1. Move to front of body. Draw Cho-Ku-Rei to open chakra
2. Hold both hands 3" (10 cm) over heart chakra & Channel the 3 symbols (4, 3 & 1)

Step 8 - Placing the three Symbols in the Hand Chakras

1. Put client's hands in prayer position; Draw Cho-Ku-Rei over them
2. Separate the hands - leave the left one in the prayer position. Hold their right hand palm facing you and draw Cho-Ku-Rei in the air over the palm whilst chanting the mantra three times. Then slap the symbol into the hand keeping your hand on theirs (as shown on the VIDEO). Then visualize a large Cho-Ku-Rei in Golden light and imprint the symbol into the hand chakra chanting the mantra three times as you do this, then remove your hand. Repeat this process with Sei-He-Kei and then again with Hon-Sha-Ze-Sho-Nen. Put their hands back in prayer position and then repeat the whole process with the other hand leaving the other hand in the prayer position. When finished bring both hands back together in the prayer position.

Step 9 - Blowing the Breath of Life and Filling the Aura

1. Draw a large Cho-Ku-Rei over solar plexus and sacral chakra (belly). Beam energy to that chakra holding the energy in that place with your hands.
2. Draw a Cho-Ku-Rei with the tip of your tongue at the top of your upper teeth on the roof of your mouth and then blow it into the solar plexus and up the body. This step b) is optional.
3. Wrap both your hands gently around their hands and blow a Cho-Ku-Rei into their Heart chakra across the tips of their fingers. Move their hands up so that the tips of their fingers are in line with their third eye and blow a Cho-Ku-Rei into the third eye. Move their hands up so that the tips of their fingers are in line with their crown and blow a Cho-Ku-Rei into the crown. Put their hands back down in original prayer position in front of their heart chakra to finish.

Step 10 - Grounding the client

Draw a large Cho-Ku-Rei over aura in front of the heart to ground them. Indicate that the hands can come down in their laps and they can open their eyes in their own time

Optional Finish after attunement

The test for Reiki 1 and 2 below allows your client to feel their Reiki energy as demonstrated on Video.

1. After the client is fully present ask them to hold their hands vertically, palms facing each other about 6" apart with their fingers pointing at you. Both hands are about level with the solar plexus or whatever is comfortable for them. You are going to test their sensitivity by bringing your hand slowly between theirs starting from about two feet away from their hands. Ask them now to close their eyes and tell you when they can feel your energy as your hand moves closer between theirs. When the client says "Now" keep your hand still. Ask them to open their eyes so they can see how close your hand is to their energy field. Then you can play in-between their hands in their energy field and ask them how it feels?

2. Now ask them to close their eyes again and to switch their Reiki on and put their hands over their eyes until they can feel the Reiki energy. When they have done this ask them "How did it feel to you?"

Reiki Master 3rd Degree Attunement

Step 1 - Opening the Aura

Draw a Large Cho-Ku-Rei over the Heart Chakra and Body

1. Ask the receiver to close their eyes before you start and then smooth down their aura.
2. Draw a large Cho-Ku-Rei over the heart chakra at the front of body to open the aura.
3. Beam Reiki healing energy to the heart area and front of body; this helps to open the heart chakra and the whole aura.

Step 2 – Right or Left Hand on Right or Left Shoulder - Other Hand Draws 3 Symbols in the air invoking Divine Chakra channelling

Walk (to your right) anticlockwise round client and place your right or left hand on their right or left shoulder and as you do this draw the 3 symbols in the air chanting their mantras 3 times using your left or right hand in the following order; Dai-Ko-Myo, Hon-Sha-Ze-Sho-Nen & Cho-Ku-Rei.

Step 3 - Opening the Crown Chakra

1. Draw a small Cho-Ku-Rei over the crown to open the chakra
2. Cup your hands over the crown and channel the 3 symbols (4, 3 & 1) down through the whole body. (Visualize the symbols in Golden light and chant their mantra three times silently as you channel each symbol into the crown.)

Step 4 Both hands on shoulders to prepare opening the heart Chakra

1. Place both hands on shoulders, fingers on collar bone to send energy to heart.
2. Channel the 3 symbols (4, 3 & 1) down the body into the heart. This helps open and attune the lower chakras.

Step 5 - Opening the Throat Chakra

1. Walk (to your right) anticlockwise to side of their body stopping in line with their shoulders and open throat with Cho-Ku-Rei. Place one hand in front and one hand at back of their throat (both hands approx. 3" - 10 cm off the body)
2. Channel the 3 symbols (4, 3 & 1)

Step 6 - Opening The Third Eye Chakra

1. Draw Cho-Ku-Rei to open third eye and then place one hand on Third eye and one hand at back of head cupping just up from the base (Near T1 Medulla Oblongata)
2. Channel the 3 symbols (4, 3 & 1) - Into third eye - Inside head between your two hands

Step 7 - Opening The Heart Chakra

1. Move to front of body. Draw Cho-Ku-Rei to open chakra
2. Hold both hands 3" (10 cm) over heart chakra and Channel the 3 symbols (4, 3 & 1)

Step 8 - Placing the Master Symbol in the Hand Chakras

1. Put client's hands in prayer position and Draw Cho-Ku-Rei over them.
2. Separate the hands - leave their left hand in the prayer position. Hold the right hand palm facing you and draw Dai-Ko-Myo in the air over the palm whilst chanting the mantra three times then slap the symbol into the hand (as shown on the VIDEO). Then visualize a large Dai-Ko-Myo in Golden light and imprint the symbol into the hand chakra, chanting the mantra again three times as you do this, then remove your hand. Put their hands back in prayer position and then repeat the whole process with the left hand leaving the right hand in the prayer position. When finished bring both hands back together in the prayer position.

Step 9 - Blowing the Breath of Life & Filling the Aura

1. Draw a large Cho-Ku-Rei over solar plexus and sacral chakra (belly). Beam energy to that chakra holding the energy in that place with your hands.
2. Draw a Cho-Ku-Rei with the tip of your tongue at the top of your upper teeth on the roof of your mouth and then blow it into the solar plexus and up the body. This step b) is optional.
3. Wrap both your hands gently around their hands and blow a Cho-Ku-Rei into their Heart chakra across the tips of their fingers. Move their hands up so that the tips of their fingers are in line with their third eye and blow a Cho-Ku-Rei into the third eye. Move their hands up so that the tips of their fingers are in line with their crown and blow a Cho-Ku-Rei into the crown. Put their hands back down in original prayer position in front of their heart chakra to finish.

Step 10 - Grounding the client

Draw a large Cho-Ku-Rei over aura in front of the heart to ground them. Indicate that the hands can come down in their laps and they can open their eyes in their own time

Optional Finish after the Attunement

The Reiki Master Attunement - Finish with the Reiki Hug as demonstration on the tutorial Video. After client is fully present ask them to stand up and both bring your heart chakras together as you hug each other allowing the Reiki Master energy to flow as you embrace. This normally is a very warm feeling.

Lesson Plan Examples

One Day Reiki First Degree

10.00am	Breathing Meditation with music start Self-Healing Heart and Solar Plexus and Induce Group Reiki Healing
10.15am	Introductions: All students and myself
10. 30am	Practical information, any questions from manual. Explain about receiving Reiki Attunements and prepare student for the Attunement; remove jewellery etc.
11.00am	Explain and practice Western and Japanese Self-Healing with their different Hand positions Form circle on floor on blankets or on chairs and begin self-healing. Practice self-healing hand positions and start healing (Begin Students Attunements whilst students are practicing their self healing, both methods)
12.00am	Refreshment Break
12.30pm	21 Day Journal - Healing Self, Family, Animals, Plants and Objects Aura Scanning and The Chakras (Practice on each other)
1.00pm	Lunch
2.00pm	Laughing Buddha Meditation or similar (if time)

2.10pm	Set up Treatment Couch - Demonstrate how to give a full Reiki Healing treatment to another person. **Key teaching point**: Healing follows the Chakra points on the body, plus the student can use whatever hand position is comfortable to them as an individual – the sequence is not set in stone as it is only a guide. Start on chair, how to treat client face down and then laying face up, add in Aura Scanning.
2.30pm	Putting it all together - Students Practice Full 50 min Reiki treatment on each other – 10 min Student Brief feedback
3.30pm	Refreshment Break
4.00pm	Full 50 min Reiki treatment – 10 min Student Brief feedback
5.00pm	Group Feedback
5.20pm	Reiki Circle to close
5.30pm	Finish

Two Day Reiki First Degree
Day One

10.00am	Breathing Meditation with music - Start Self-Healing Heart and Solar Plexus and Induce Group Reiki Healing
10.15am	Select an Angel Card– Impressions – colour etc. Introductions: All students and yourself (Place Angel Cards or whatever you wish to use, at altar area for course duration, review at end of course if time) *This introduction is optional and is in accordance with your own beliefs*
10. 30am	Practical information, any questions from manual. Explain about receiving 3 Reiki Attunements and prepare student for the Attunement; remove jewellery etc.
11.00am	Explain Western and Japanese Self-Healing with their 5 Hand positions. Form circle on floor on blankets or chairs and begin self healing. Practice self healing hand positions and start practice (Begin Students' First Attunement)
12.00am	Refreshment Break
12.30pm	21 Day Journal - Aura Scanning with Energy sensing (Practice on each other)
1.00pm	Lunch & Walk
2.30pm	Laughing Buddha or Similar to bring group back to focus

2.40pm	Explain the Chakras and how Reiki is used for Physical, Emotional and Mental Healing. (Brings all back to balance) Reiki Well-Being exercise - Instructions for 5 hand positions Form circle on floor on blankets or chairs and begin self healing (Begin Students' Second Attunement)
3.30pm	Refreshment Break
4.00pm	Demonstrate Full Reiki Treatment on a chair – 8 Positions
4.15pm	Students exchange practice 25 min Reiki treatment on a chair Allow 3 min feedback one to one
5.25pm	Reiki Circle to close
5.30pm	Finish

Two Day Reiki First Degree
Day Two

10.00am	Aura soma cleanse - Meditation – Self empowerment
10.15am	Feedback any impressions, experiences, insights
10.30am	Self Healing (students choice) – Start Third Initiation Attunement
11.30am	Refreshment Break
12.00am	Explain how the Chakras relate to the Reiki Healing hand positions in all treatments. Couch Demonstration - Aura Scanning and how to treat the client face down – 5 hand positions

12.15pm	Students exchange practice on each other, face down treatment (allow 2 min for each hand position) One to one 3 min feedback
1.00pm	Lunch & Walk
2.30pm	Demonstrate on treatment couch how to give a treatment to another person laying face up (10 hand positions)
2.45pm	Students exchange practice on each other, face up treatment (allow 3 min for each hand position) One to one 3 min feedback
3.50pm	Refreshment Break
4.20pm	Putting it all together (This exercise is to prove knowledge of hand position healing sequence, not a Reiki treatment exercise. Students monitor and help each other in this exercise). Students practice full sequence on each other. Starting on a chair, onto the couch to treat the back and then turning over to treat the front of the body – Allow 3 min one to one feedback
5.00pm	The Uses of Reiki Healing: People, Animals, Plants and Objects, Questions and Answers
5.25pm	Reiki Circle - Meditation on 'I am Love' to close
5.30pm	Finish

Two Day Reiki Second Degree
Day One

10.00am	Reiki Circle & Angel card with Introductions All students & myself
10.30am	Sound & Vibration – Nadabrahma Meditation
10.50am	Difference between Western and Japanese use of Symbols Key Teaching point: Chanting the mantras will invoke them allowing you to become one with the energy Reminder of Aura Scanning and Self Scanning Student practice self Aura Scanning with self healing while Students receive Second Degree Reiki Attunements
11.30am	Refreshment Break
12.00am	Cho-Ku-Rei – Physical - Best use hands on body Use to open, close and grounding Drawing symbol and Chanting mantra energy
12.30pm	Student exchange treatment Aura scanning with Cho-Ku-Rei
1.00pm	Lunch and Walk
2.30pm	Ayurveda –Different stress tolerances for 3 personality types Learn Patience and Tolerance – Non Judgemental Mind Love and Acceptance of Self and Others
2.50pm	Sei-Hei-Ki – Best use hands off body Emotional intelligence - The Heart Chakra Drawing symbol and Chanting mantra energy

3.20pm	Student exchange treatment Chakra Balancing with Sei-Hei-Ki
4.00pm	Refreshment Break
4.30pm	Student exchange treatment – All chakras Chakra Balancing with Sei-Hei-Ki and Cho-Ku-Rei
5.20pm	Reiki Circle to close
5.30pm	Finish off day 1

Two Day Reiki Second Degree
Day Two

10.00am	Reiki Circle and Loving Kindness Meditation on Unity
10.30am	Day 1 and last night feedback – Impressions and experiences
10.50am	Radiating Beauty from Loving Kindness Oneness of Life
11.00am	Hon-Sha-Ze-Sho-Nen – Mind and Distant Healing Drawing symbol and Chanting mantra energy
11.30am	Refreshment Break
12.00am	Intention – How Reiki will follow your intention Beaming – Hands, Eyes, Heart and Breath Student exchange treatment in same room Beaming with Hon-Sha-Ze-Sho-Nen
12.25pm	Manifesting your desires – The creation of life's ambitions Explain how to heal the inner child with Hon-Sha-Ze-Sho-Nen Distant Healing with Hon-Sha-Ze-Sho-Nen Healing the Inner Child Student exchange treatment in different locations
1.00pm	Lunch
2.30pm	Introduce 'The practice of Respect' self and client, all of life The Practice of Gratitude – relief from dissatisfaction Student exchange treatments Putting it all together 40 min professional treatment
4.00pm	Refreshment Break

4.30pm	Feedback with any Questions and Answers Running a Professional Practice
5.00pm	Combination Meditation; Reiki, Breathing and Self-empowerment visualisation - I am Love
5.20pm	Reiki Circle to close
5.30pm	Finish

One Day Reiki Master

10.00am	Reiki Circle and Welcome
10.30am	Chanting The Lotus Sutra Mantra for Master's Wisdom
11.00am	Give student course handbook and review contents Draw 'The Masters Symbol' become familiar with it
11.30am	Refreshment Break
12.00am	Sound and Vibration – Chanting The Reiki Master's Mantra Dai-Ko-Myo Feedback of experience
12.30pm	Lunch
2.30pm	Combination Meditation; Breathing with Reiki Self-empowerment visualisation – I am Love
2.45pm	Reiki Master Attunements
3.30pm	Refreshment Break
4.00pm	Questions and Answers - Discussion
4.30pm	Reiki Circle and Loving kindness Meditation on Unity
5.00pm	Finish

Meditations and Self Help Exercises

KEY EXERCISE TO AWAKEN THE THREE REIKI ENERGIES

Chant the Mantra of each energy until you become one with it

Take one energy at a time starting with Cho-Ku-Rei. Draw the symbol three times and chant the mantra for as long as you require, enabling you to feel the powerful Reiki energy manifesting in your whole being; until you become one with the energy. You can stop chanting as soon as you can feel the energy in your body - this could be for a period of ten minutes up to one-hour duration. As soon as you are completely happy you are one with the energy, stop chanting, close your eyes and enjoy the experience. Go into it; merge yourself with the feelings and sensations of being one with Cho-Ku-Rei. It is good to deepen your experience with Cho-Ku-Rei by repeating this exercise everyday for at least three days.

The key teaching points

- To make this experience permanent is to allow a minimum period of three days before you start working with Sei-Hei-Ki and the same with Hon-Sha-Ze-Sho-Nen.

- The reason for this is probably obvious but it is important to deepen your relationship with Cho-Ku-Rei before attempting to become one with Sei-Hei-Ki.

- Three days are an important period of time because this will enable your whole being to process the experience making it a learnt permanent memory within your life.

- Repeat the above exercise with Sei-Hei-Ki and then with Hon-Sha-Ze-Sho-Nen.

TRANSFORMING PAIN INTO LOVE

If both expressing and holding back negative feelings can be harmful what should you do when the emotions boil up in you? The moment the emotion comes up look into it, embrace it and then introduce Sei-Hei-Ki. When you do this exercise look at the feeling or emotion without labeling it.

When the heart closes the soul energy returns to the mind and solar plexus; you have fallen in consciousness and have become trapped within your lower human self. When this happens you experience pain and suffering with all the negative emotions and negative fearful thoughts that accompany this experience of life. There is a very simple solution, introduce love through your heart chakra using Sei-Hei-Ki. Self healing is very powerful when you use Sei-Hei-Ki to open your heart chakra to feel and experience love once again; feeling peacefully at ease.

Let's suppose it is a feeling of anger. Take a long deep breath, let yourself feel the anger and exhale. This will help. You can then draw the emotional symbol over your solar plexus chakra and place one hand over it with the other hand placed over your heart chakra; this will have the effect of bringing love to your heart chakra and bring harmony back to your ego felt in the solar plexus. This energy is felt more powerfully if the hands are held about three inches off the body.

You will experience a release as the heart chakra opens and your mind will become calm once again. If you felt the anger as a result of a relationship conflict it will dissolve and transform and the other person will also calm down.

You allow the feeling to be what it is, giving it total freedom to express itself. You have to be aware of the external energy information input, for example what your partner or friend is saying, as well as at the same time bringing awareness to what is happening inside of you. When awareness goes both ways inner and outer, understanding is then totally experienced. The emotion now becomes expressed and realized, being lived in the present moment and not repressed. It is repression that creates disease.

USING SEI-HEI-KI IN REIKI TREATMENTS

As Sei-Hei-Ki is the feminine receptive heavenly unconditional love energy, the emotional intelligence, it is most effective when it is drawn over the brow Chakra, the heart Chakra and the Solar Plexus

Use the following positive affirmations with this symbol:-

- You are calm, content and serene
- You are loved and secure
- You are safe
- You feel loved and are lovable - I am love, you are love

The same approach is used as in the exercise 'Transforming Pain into Love'. If both expressing and holding back negative feelings can be harmful what should you do when the emotions boil up in you? The moment the emotion comes up look into it.

Let's suppose it is a feeling of anger you wish to transform

- Take a long deep breath. Let yourself feel the anger and exhale. This will help.

- You can then draw Sei-Hei-Ki the emotional symbol over your solar plexus chakra and place one hand over it and the other hand over your heart chakra; this will have the effect of bringing love to your heart chakra and bring harmony back to your ego felt in the solar plexus.

- You will experience a release as the heart chakra opens and your mind will become calm once again.

- If the anger you felt was as a result of a relationship conflict, it will melt and the other person will also calm down.

You allow the feeling 'total freedom' to express itself. You have to be aware not only of the external energy information input, for example what your partner or friend is saying but at the same time you have to bring awareness to your inner-self.

When awareness goes both ways inner and outer understanding is then totally experienced. The emotion now becomes expressed and realized, being lived in the present moment and not repressed. It is repression that creates disease.

When you do this exercise look at the feeling or emotion without labeling it.

CREATING BALANCE BETWEEN THE EMOTIONAL AND THE PHYSICAL

Activate your Reiki energy using Cho-Ku-Rei. Then place the Sei-Hei-Ki symbol over the following three chakras: the brow or third eye sixth chakra, the heart fourth chakra and the sacral second chakra.

The reason these three chakras have been selected is because they tend to be more receptive than expressive as their function is to connect the emotional body with the physical body and the Divine spiritual body. Any emotional blockages at a level of unconscious awareness will be released and balanced creating healing.

As you have learnt, Reiki comes from Unconditional Love connecting and balancing the emotional body and will result in every cell in your physical body expressing wellness and health. With repeated healing sessions emotions will start becoming heart felt.

When you experience a heart felt emotion your emotional body has become connected to your spirit, enabling you to live your life with joy in each moment of your experience; your subtle senses have touched a specific area within your spiritual body. This subtle sense of touch actually does feel at a level beyond the physical sensation.

Nature has given us these three inner chakras, these extensions of touch, to enable us to feel how another person feels at an unconscious level, connecting our emotional bodies with theirs. At a more subtle level you will learn to feel the finer aspects of emotion where every day feelings get purified into love, devotion and compassion. At the very threshold of pure awareness where all emotions dissolve into bliss you can contact every aspect of refined emotion where you actually experience the slightest impulse of love as complete fulfillment.

NEW AWAKENING METHOD FOR DISTANT HEALING

How to activate Hon-Sha-Ze-Sho-Nen

When working in the spiritual plane, centre yourself, which is just another way of saying get into a comfortable position and activate Reiki. Close your eyes, take a long deep breath and let your thoughts wander where they will (just let go of your mind).

1. **Preparation** - Visualize or draw Cho-Ku-Rei over your feet to anchor you in the here and now, the physical body.

2. **Preparation** - Visualize or draw Sei-Hei-Ki over your heart chakra to centre your emotional body in Love.

3. **Activate Distant Healing** - Visualize or draw Hon-Sha-Ze-Sho-Nen in your mind and state your request. If you want to go back to a certain period in time that is what you ask for.

For example, if you have had a previous physical problem you would request the following 'to go back in your mind to the time exactly when the situation occurred.' Stating your destination tells your consciousness where to stop. It is a subtle feeling but you know when you have reached the particular time period. When you are conscious of that past time you acknowledge a new situation; that you have a perfectly healthy body, enjoy good health and that you are aware your body is working perfectly.

You then visualize the Hon-Sha-Ze-Sho-Nen symbol again and ask to be brought back to the present time with your body in this completely new healthy state.

HEALING YOURSELF AND OTHERS THROUGH THE SPIRITUAL PLANE

As your capacity for compassion expands, your heart becomes more open. Your capacity to bear the pain of others will become more noticeable. Your friends, clients and family will come to you unconsciously for healing even without their deliberate intention. You will feel their emotional body in yourself, there will be an ability to experience what they are experiencing without knowing the details of their circumstances. This is the development of Unconditional Love, of Oneness.

I have noticed that I can be perfectly happy and for no reason I can start to feel uncomfortable in myself. This is sometimes experienced as emotional pain in the solar plexus or experienced as tension or fuzziness in my third eye. No one is communicating with me directly but am I feeling the pain of someone whom I know on the inner spiritual planes?

The solution to this experience is very simple; to send distance healing to yourself and whoever is unconsciously calling on you for healing, even though you do not know who it may be. When I do this I also add the emotional symbol Sei-Hei-Ki to send love to everyone who is in need of healing, including myself.

Imagine the Other Person and Yourself between your Hands

- Prepare yourself for distant healing using Cho-Ku-Rei and Sei-Hei-Ki.
- Hold your hands apart and start your distant healing.
- Now using your intention send the healing for the benefit of whoever is in need of healing. (Remember you do not know).
- The main person to include is yourself because in some way you are karmically involved in the situation.
- Now add the emotional symbol of Love. (You can also chant the mantra of 'I Love You').
- Hold the energy until you feel comfort return to your mind or body.

INNER CHILD HEALING

This method of healing yourself through Hon-Sha-Ze-Sho-Nen using the spiritual planes is also used to heal the inner child inside of you. This is a very powerful way to heal your past childhood. We all have many past hurts and misunderstandings learnt in our childhood which can limit our lives as adults.

Imagine yourself as a child and hold your inner child between your hands and send the symbols as your hands transmit Reiki. You can ask the Reiki to repeat the healing session every half-hour for 24 hours. Chanting the symbols' names is a very powerful way to increase the Reiki energy level.

Imagine your Inner Child between your Hands

- Prepare yourself for distant healing using Cho-Ku-Rei and Sei-Hei-Ki.
- Hold your hands apart and start your distant healing.
- Now using your intention send the healing to your inner child.
- Now add the emotional symbol of Love. (You can also chant the mantra of 'I Love You')
- Hold the energy until you feel comfort return to your mind or body.

THE ROSE METHOD
FOR SENDING DISTANT HEALING

One method is to create a rose. Being on the internet and belonging to many healing groups, I receive regular healing requests. As I receive each request, I print them out for my convenience. When I have a pile of requests, I sit down, relax, put my hands on the pile and close my eyes. I first of all establish a strong Reiki energy using Cho-Ku-Rei. I then mentally ask each of the recipients if they will accept a Reiki healing, adding that if someone does not desire the healing it would go to someone who wants and needs it.

I then visualize a rosebud and mentally draw Hon-Sha-Ze-Sho-Nen superimposed over the rose bud. This has the effect of opening a spiritual pathway the healing energy will take to connect with the recipients.

I state my request that this healing energy will be delivered to each of the names on the list and request that the healing energy is to repeat every half hour for 24 hours.

I then send the healing by mentally drawing the Hon-Sha-Ze-Sho-Nen again while I watch the rose in my imagination slowly open. When the rose is fully open I thank the Divine by saying, "And so it is." I open my eyes knowing everyone on the list has received a healing session.

To finish the healing session I close with a Cho-Ku-Rei.

USING THE ROSE METHOD IN A HEALING GROUP

At the close of a Reiki exchange night everyone sits in a circle and I guide the group through a long distance healing session. I have everyone close his or her eyes and picture a rose bud. I ask everyone there to anchor themselves in Cho-Ku-Rei and Sei-Hei-Ki and then to visualize the Hon-Sha-Ze-Sho-Nen symbol.

Anyone who has a healing request now says the names out loud. I wait until everybody has stated his or her healing requests.

Then I request this energy be directed to those who are willing to accept it and if they are not that the energy goes to someone who wants and needs it. I ask the Reiki to repeat the session every half-hour for 24 hours.

I then ask all the Reiki practitioners to visualize Hon-Sha-Ze-Sho-Nen. Next I ask everyone to see the rose-bud opening knowing that when it is fully open the healing sessions will be sent. Again I thank the Divine; draw a Cho-Ku-Rei and have everyone open his or her eyes. The energy level in the room is phenomenal.

CHAKRA BALANCING

It is a good idea to revise the section on 'The Chakras' as taught on the Reiki First Degree course. This chakra balancing technique becomes most effective with the hands several inches (4 to 6) above the physical body. You will soon discover what the best distance from the body is by finding the centre of the energy chakra. This point is where you feel that the energy is at its strongest (always have the palms of your hands facing the clients body).

1. Place one hand above the brow or third eye chakra and the other hand above the root chakra.
2. Wait until you have the same feeling in both hands and establish a balance between both areas feeling the Reiki energy flowing.
3. Move the hand down from the brow sixth chakra to the throat fifth chakra and at the same time move the hand up from the root first chakra to the sacral second chakra.
4. Move the hand down from the throat chakra to the heart fourth chakra and at the same time move the hand up from the sacral second chakra to the solar plexus third chakra.

Do not hurry over the chakras; just take your time and feel with your intuition the changes in the energy centres and wait for the balance to be established. This is a very powerful technique because it rebalances each individual chakra back to functioning in its positive mode.

We normally find that the lower body does not have enough energy owing to the fact that we tend to live too much in our minds as a result of our western society.

The crown chakra is divinely connected therefore it has an unlimited supply of universal energy and does not require balancing.

When performing chakra balancing it is best to treat the front of the body. This balancing exercise can be done at the end of a hands-on Reiki session or as a short treatment on its own.

These exercises can be incorporated into another therapy as an additional tool. In all the exercises above it is a good idea to smooth the aura to finish the treatment.

Avoid using your mind and making judgements. Just allow the Reiki to flow naturally when it is being drawn into any particular chakra. The client's body and spirit will take the Reiki where it needs healing nourishment.

You can also balance chakras one at a time

OBSERVING YOUR RELATIONSHIPS

Developing Loving Kindness to yourself and others

Notice any negative thoughts or feelings that you turn inwards towards yourself or that are projected outwards towards other people.

1. Interrupt them instantly and chant Cho-Ku-Rei at least three times. This will activate Reiki and bring a higher energy to the moment. When you are chanting (if this is possible) you can place one hand over your heart and one over your solar plexus.
2. When you feel that you have interrupted the old pattern then mentally direct to yourself, or the other person, the practice of respect: "I deeply respect your life".

The interesting point is that just by bringing awareness to a situation, by inviting the Divine Healing energy into that moment of your life, transformation occurs. This is the beginning in a course of miracles. More deeply rooted unwanted patterns will be dealt with on a latter course and it is a good idea to record anything you want to change in your journal. You are now preparing the foundation for your spiritual freedom.

It is very important to record in your journal any positive changes you notice or positive remarks that are made to you by other people: for example "you appear a little calmer these days", "There is something different about you but I can't put my finger on what it is". Write down any colours you experienced on your Reiki attunement, new sensations, vivid dreams, or impressions you have experienced, no matter how small they may appear.

THE PRACTICE OF CHANTING 'I LOVE YOU'

Your main Goal in life should be 'Spiritual Awakening' which is a state of inner indestructible Happiness. You then discover that the limits in your life are only your own!

At the core of everyone - YOU and I and everyone else, we all want love. When you say or chant 'I Love You' as a mantra inside of yourself, you cleanse yourself of negative emotions and radiate at your core energy, which is LOVE.

You then RADIATE an energy that is common to us all and everyone feels it. The result is everything comes to you!

Chant or repeatedly say

'I Love You' 'I Love You' 'I Love You'

Repeat this mantra until you can feel a change inside of you

Use this mantra to Love your worries, problems, blocks, illness and they will transform into the Universal core energy of Unconditional Love. Mix this practice with the practice of Gratitude to increase its power. Connect with Reiki and start chanting the mantra to deepen your experience.

THE LOVING KINDNESS MEDITATION

"May all beings be well
May they be free from suffering
May all beings find their Divine light"

By connecting with your underlying nature you will discover an awareness of pure love. Do this repeatedly until the heart exhibits its true nature. In the meantime it is skilful to cultivate such feelings as loving kindness towards all living beings.

Paradoxically the cultivation of loving kindness through meditation and daily practice is almost like using the water drill in order to hit the water table below, releasing the enormous rivers of compassion and mercy which lay just below the surface of our ever active mind.

In an odd way the necessary cultivation of such qualities as loving kindness and sympathetic joy are almost an imitation of our essential nature. The fears then disintegrate and the love grows greater.

Stephen Levine

The love you seek is seeking you at this moment

Be kind to yourself and others
Come from love every moment you can
Speak of others with love
Remind each other of your spiritual purpose
Never give up hope
Know that you are loved

THE PRACTICE OF GRATITUDE

Gratitude and acknowledgement are essential components in attracting whatever you want in your life. Practicing gratitude eliminates personal dissatisfaction and complaining. This exercise will deepen the power, influence and effect of the exercise of chanting 'I LOVE YOU'.

Through the expression of gratitude on a daily basis you will create an even greater vibrational match for the future you want to create.

We recommend that you practice gratitude in the following way:

First take a deep breath, become centered so that you pay attention to your second sacral chakra (just below your belly button). This will bring focus and depth to what you are about to be grateful for.

Then say, with passion and emotional meaning, "I am grateful for ...." list as many as possible.

When you have finished this exercise just sit with as empty a mind as possible and notice how you feel emotionally.

The importance of keeping a Gratitude Journal

(The importance of keeping the journal – You can then go back and read from it and add new things to be grateful for. The journal will also reveal the spiritual growth of an individual as more human elements such as "I am grateful for my mother – I am grateful for my father – I am grateful for my boss" will emerge as a person develops more compassion, moving from things for me to social considerations).

BREATHING MEDITATION

Breathing exercise to induce the Alpha state

Deep breathing from the diaphragm is the key to relaxation. A full deep breath increases the amount of oxygen as the body begins to function effectively, especially during mental activity.

To feel the full effect of correct breathing, place your hand over your navel and imagine you have a balloon in your stomach. Breathe deeply through the nose - as the balloon inflates your hand moves outwards. As you breathe out imagine the balloon deflating and feel the abdomen falling.

Before starting any exercise on relaxation always take three full deep breaths - and feel the tension and negative energy drain away on the out breath, breathing in positive energy on the in breath. Once you have learnt this breathing method to achieve meditation try using it with your Reiki Self Healing.

Here is the simple procedure

1. Imagine the balloon in your abdomen as this is where you transfer your consciousness. Breathe in relaxation and positive energy and hold the breath for three seconds.

2. Breathe out letting go of any tension and negative energy - feel the balloon deflate - and again hold the breath for three seconds. Become aware of the precise moment of stillness.

3. Breathe in again - be aware of the air filling your lungs - hold for three seconds.

4. Breathe out with a sigh - feel the air leaving your body. Hold for three seconds.

5. Breathe in - be aware of the air flowing in. Hold for three seconds.

6. Breathe out with a sigh and feel the tension draining away.

CREATING A POSITIVE SELF-IMAGE

When you are experiencing negative feelings about yourself the following exercise will help you regain a positive self image of yourself. This will have a knock on effect of re establishing your positive sense of self worth.

1. When you feel good about yourself your life condition will increase. What is happening? You are once again opening your heart to allow your higher loving self to transform your negative emotions into love. When you are really stuck and are unable to start this exercise because you feel so negative, use your Reiki healing to help lift you.

2. Imagine yourself as you would ideally like to be. Think about how you would look if you were as happy and confident as you wanted to be. How would you walk? What would you wear? What expressions are on your face? Where do you go? Take as much time as you need to see how you look when you are confident and full of self-esteem.

3. When you know what you will look like, make a little movie clip in your imagination of yourself, happy, confident and self-assured.

4. Now, imagine stepping into yourself in that movie. See what you see, hear what you hear and feel the confidence of being there and enjoying being exactly how you want to be.

5. Imagine waking up tomorrow as your ideal self feeling this good and imagine the day going exactly as you want it to.

6. Start your Reiki energy and then using your imagination send the Reiki energy to the new you.

In order to get a maximum benefit from this technique, please use it daily for at least a week. Keep on using for longer up to 21 days, or as often as you want to.

DEVELOPING SELF LOVE AND APPRECIATION

This is another exercise that will help you to feel better about yourself. It will also have the effect of re-establishing your self-respect and self-love. Whenever you are feeling low, depressed or are self-doubting it is your cherished friends and family who can see your strengths and values when you cannot. They will offer you affection, acceptance, appreciation and most importantly Love. When you see yourself as they can see you, your thoughts and feelings about yourself will transform into Self-Love.

1. Take several deep breaths to centre you and close your eyes. For about five minutes use the breathing meditation whilst at the same time also give yourself Reiki healing. Hold one hand over your heart chakra and the other hand over your solar plexus chakra.
2. Now think of someone who loves or deeply appreciates you. Remember how they look and imagine that they are standing in front of you.
3. Imagine stepping out of your body and into the body of the person who loves you. See through their eyes, hear through their ears and feel their love and good feelings as they look at you.
4. Notice in detail what it is that they appreciate about you. Finally understand these amazing qualities that perhaps you haven't appreciated about yourself until now. Take a few moments to feel good as you look at yourself.
5. Notice where the feeling is the strongest and give it a colour.
6. Imagine spreading that colour all through you, up to the top of your head and down to the tips of your toes.
7. Now double its intensity and brightness, deepening the energy in your imagination.
8. As you open your eyes keep that feeling glowing inside you.

You can keep that inner feeling with you for hours and hours and repeat this exercise whenever you want to boost it. The more you do it, the easier it becomes and eventually it becomes automatic to love and feel loved.

The Dalai Lama apparently cried when he discovered that Western people had difficulty in loving themselves because from his Buddhist culture the idea of loving yourself is part of their conditioning.

THE LAUGHING BUDDHA

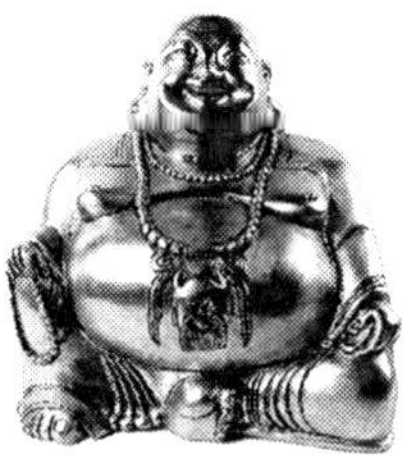

Hotei was a wandering monk who went around and took the sadness from people of this world. Due to his large protruding stomach and his smile, he is known as the Laughing Buddha. In China, he is dubbed the Loving or Friendly One. His image graces many temples, restaurants and amulets. Hotei has become a deity of contentment and abundance. Hotei shows us the power of laughter to transform our attitude towards life. He used it as a spiritual practice for himself and other people and it worked!

Laughter has more importance in transforming us than we realise; try feeling miserable when you are laughing. Today there are Laughter Therapists to lift people with depression and help transform the negative emotions that cause illness. People have just become well through the practice of laughter.

In our lives we tend to get caught up, stuck in the troubles and problems of everyday life at the expense of the beautiful richness contained within us; the higher self waiting to lift us into love to experience the sheer joy of existence.

Laughter is infectious - Become like Hotei then more homes will be full of laughter, dancing and singing. Lose your seriousness and you will become more healthy and whole. Enjoy this simple, fun exercise. I promise you it really does work. Your laughter will spread, it will become infectious so that tidal waves of laughter will spread everywhere. Your laughter will bring a gift of such joy and celebration to everyone. Explore it, enjoy it, most of all lighten up and have fun.

The Laughing Buddha Exercise

- This exercise will help you to laugh for no reason at all. If you can laugh early in the morning then laughter will come easily throughout the day and it will lead to more laughter.

- Do this technique between five and ten minutes, with eyes open or closed on your own or in a group. It is great for breaking through the awkwardness of social politeness, especially when people meet for the first time. This will create openness within any group, bringing humanness, love and warmth.

- After a minute or two start to laugh. Simply lift the corners of your mouth and laugh, even if you do not feel like it. Soon forced laughter stimulates the real thing and your laughter will become quite spontaneous. This will change the mood of your whole day.

THE PRACTICE OF RESPECT

This very simple spiritual practice will bring amazing changes to your state of being.

Try it. Silently greet every person you meet 3 times with "I deeply respect your life".

Try this even if you do not appreciate the other person. What you are doing is greeting their life as a spiritual being, on a level that is beyond judgement. You are raising your vibration to a new greeting of 'The God in me recognizes and honors the God in you; Namaste'. You will experience benefit as a result.

CHANGING NEGATIVE INTERNAL DIALOGUE

Whenever you find yourself using your inner voice to talk about your situation in a negative way, listen to the voice that you can hear, remembering what it sounds like and then create a new voice to talk to yourself. The difference is that this new voice will be positive and will talk to you in way to make you feel better about yourself; it will be on your side.

You can still hear exactly the same words and learn from whatever you are thinking but there is no need to feel bad unnecessarily! You are going to be creative and using the new voice you are going to say positive things to yourself to make you feel good about yourself. A good way to find a better form of words is to ask yourself how you would talk to a younger person whom you were helping to deal with a problem. Therefore instead of cursing or nagging yourself, try using kinder and more encouraging words to guide you towards what you want.

- I want you now to think of the last time that you used your inner voice to talk to yourself or others. Remember what you were saying to yourself; remember the specific sentence you used, or type of statement you would have said to yourself.
- Repeat the statement that you made to yourself but change the tone of voice. Keep repeating exactly the same words, but make the tone of the voice different. Make it excited or happy. Make it funny or friendly. Make it sound like a cartoon character Experiment by using all sorts of different tones of voice with exactly the same words until you find a tone that makes you feel completely different and one that brings you positive feelings.
- Now choose another voice. Choose an encouraging voice, the voice of a friend or a film star, or a voice with an accent you really like. You can play your inner voice in many more ways. You can speed it up or slow it down. You can make it higher or lower.
- Keep changing it until you find the characteristics that make it friendly, supportive and most of all loving and kind.

THE FRIENDLY MIRROR

This technique was created by Michael Breen and instantly makes you feel good about how you look! You can do this any time you are in a room with a mirror. Many people condition themselves to feel bad by looking in the mirror and think about wrinkles or fat. This technique turns all that on its head and conditions you to feel happy about your appearance.

1. Sit yourself down where you can turn and look at the mirror, but don't look at it just yet.
2. Think of the time when someone you know to be sincere paid you a compliment.
3. Remember what they said and hear it again in your mind and remember how it made you feel.
4. Imagine that feeling of being complimented, loved and cherished spreading though you like ink spreading through blotting paper. The more it spreads the more powerful it gets.
5. Now turn and look at yourself in the mirror.
6. Enjoy it!
7. Finally, imagine taking a picture of yourself just like that. Imagine taking a picture right into your heart. Keep it there so that you can look at it whenever you want to remind yourself how good you feel. You can send it into the future at any time for you to step into using Hon-Sha-Ze-Sho-Nen.

Two human rights are - Self-esteem and Self-confidence

WALKING MEDITATION

Normally, when we walk the mind becomes very active; we do not even notice what the body is doing. Only when we are interrupted do we become aware of it and are thrown into the present. Walking and becoming aware of each movement is a meditation; relieving tension and calming the mind. This technique is based on the awareness of the feet touching the ground. You can walk in a circle or a straight line of ten to fifteen steps back and forth, indoors or outdoors.

Instructions (15 minutes)

- Walk slowly, with your awareness focused on your feet as they touch the ground. Keep your eyes lowered to the ground, so that you can see only a few steps ahead. If you like, place your hands on your heart centre.
- While walking pay attention to the contact of each foot as it touches the ground. As you walk in slow motion you can say, 'Right' when the right foot touches the ground and say, 'Left' when the left foot touches the ground.
- If other things arise in your mind, notice what else takes your attention and then return to your feet.

General Awareness Meditation

- Anything can become your object for witnessing. Any action, any daily routine, such as eating, washing-up, cleaning the house, talking, jogging, dancing, or reading, can become a meditation.
- Be aware of the movements and sensations of your body, while you are walking, eating, or taking a shower. Just become alert. The meditation can enrich the quality of everyday life.

Appendix

Books, Websites and Music Source

The music of Deva Premal and Miten

www.mitendevapremal.com	www.prabhumusic.net
Cygnus Books	www.cygnus-books.co.uk
Gaia Books Ltd. London	www.Gaiabooks.com
Reiki Magazine International	www.ReikiMagazine.com
Body & Mind Music CD Store	www.bluewatermusic.net
New World Music	www.newworldmusic.com
Music for healing, chant & dance	www.soundtravels.co.uk
Amazon Books CDs & DVDs	www.amazon.com
Spirituality - New Awakening	www.new-awakening.co.uk

Reiki Master and The Lotus Sutra - Tutorial 2 CD Album and MP3 Set

Track	Description & Page Numbers	Total Time 123 minutes
1	New Awakening Introduction	5.05
2	Reiki Master 3rd degree	4.51
3	Becoming a better healer	12.26
4	Overview of 3 Reiki degrees	5.42
5	The Masters Symbol & Mantra	2.47
6	The Loving Kindness Meditation	2.02
7	The Lotus Sutra	12.51
8	Practicing The Lotus Sutra	4.27
9	Chanting the Mantra	1.24
10	Ichinen Sanzen	15.09
11	The Tan Worlds	29.41
12	The Ten Factors	16.09
13	The Three Realms of Existence	10.48

My gift to you, a spiritual resource for the world

I have provided FREE OF CHARGE part two of your course which is the Attunement. I have also supplied FREE OF CHARGE three tutorial Videos which show you how to give Reiki Healing treatments on a couch, on a chair and how to scan the aura. Please go to our website at **www.new-awakening.co.uk** to view these videos as often as you like.

There are no restrictions as to how many times you can view these videos.

How to use the Reiki Master Degree Distant Attunement Video

1. Watch the VIDEO all the way through on your own, in a place where you won't be interrupted, to get the gist of what is going to happen. Unplug the phone etc.
2. To feel a deeper experience continue by relaxing your state of mind by doing the Breathing Meditation listed at the back of this manual. This will prepare you to attune yourself more effectively.
3. Start your Reiki Healing and then start chanting Dai-Ko-Myo to invoke the Master's energy, as it is this energy that is used to transfer the spiritual attunements.
4. Then replay the Video again from the beginning, this time taking 3 deep breaths, centre your awareness in your sacral chakra, moving your energy down from your mind. Relax and close your eyes. Now imagine that it is you sitting in the chair receiving the attunement.
5. When instructions are given, this is when I will now be talking to you and guiding you through the attunement. Following the sequence you can either do the instructed actions physically or see yourself doing them in your imagination.

Reiki Certificate of Training

Students who have studied the New Awakening Reiki System of Spiritual development qualify for a certificate of attainment. To obtain your certificate go to our website at: **www.new-awakening.co.uk** Then select 'spirituality' to see the log in area 'certificates'

You will need to log into the page: User name: **certificate** Password: **certificate**

The Complete New Awakening Spiritual System

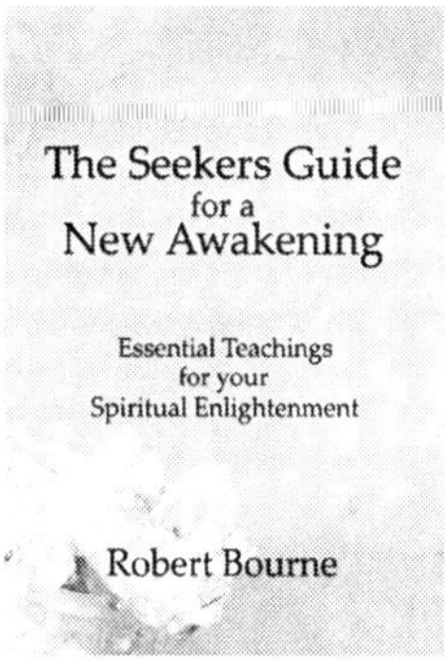

The Seekers Guide for a New Awakening

Essential Teachings for Your Spiritual Enlightenment

The Excellent You – How to get what you really want
Love and Relationships – Creating loving meaningful relationships
The Gateway to Enlightenment – Awakening to Universal Laws
Home Study Material Available
The Seekers Guide, Audio Course 6 CDs plus a Meditation CD
Includes Free Spiritual Attunements **ISBN 978-0-9561159-7-3**

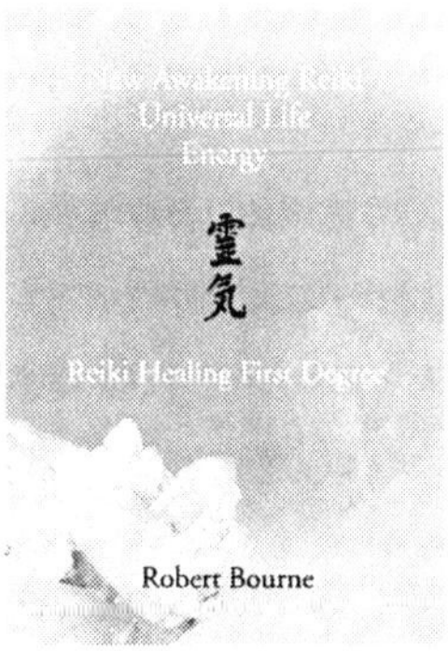

Reiki Healing First Degree New Awakening System

This Home Study Multimedia Course is all about Healing Yourself, Family, Friends, Pets and Plants
Home Study Material Available
Course Manual, Reiki Music CD, Tutorial Audio Course CDs
Includes Free Spiritual Attunements **ISBN 978-0-9561159-4-2**

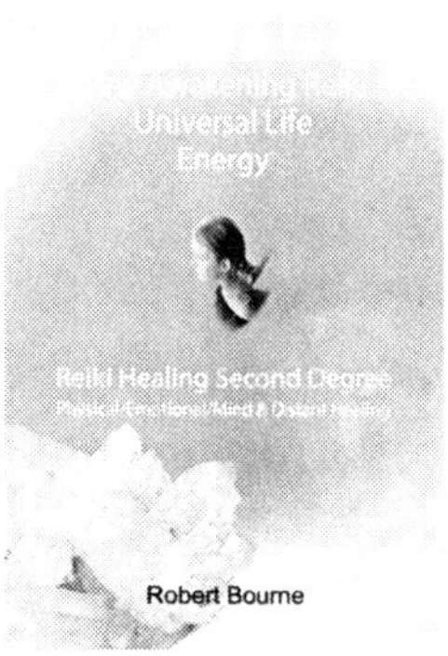

Reiki Healing Second Degree New Awakening System

This Home Study Multimedia Course Teaches Three Sacred Reiki Symbols for Physical, Emotional, Mental & Spiritual Distant Healing
Home Study Material Available
Course Manual, Reiki Music CD, Tutorial Audio Course CD set
Includes Free Spiritual Attunements **ISBN 978-0-9561159-5-9**

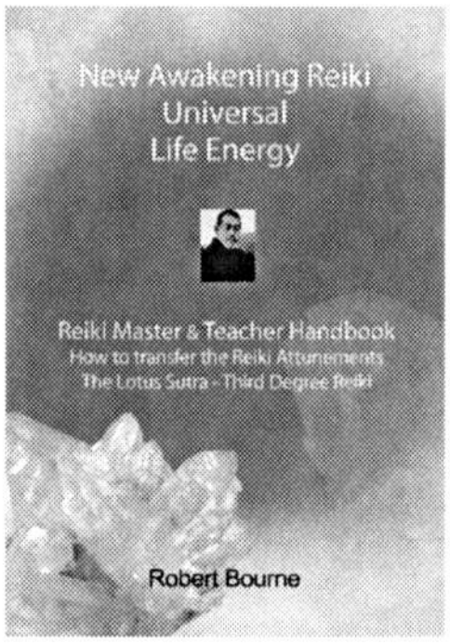

The Reiki Master – Teacher New Awakening System

This Home Study Multimedia Course Teaches
The Reiki Masters Symbol and Divine Wisdom
How to Teach Reiki & Transfer the Spiritual Attunements
Home Study Material Available
Course Book Manual, Tutorial Audio Course CD set **Includes Free Spiritual Attunements ISBN 978-0-9561159-2-8**

The 'New Awakening' method has a compassionate methodical approach through providing proven energy experiences which build upon each other creating a solid safe foundation for the student. This compassionate system created for the individual will enable the next spiritual opening to naturally occur safely. 'New Awakening' will support you with Divine Wisdom, Healing and Unconditional Love.

The 'New Awakening' system also provides three wisdom based companion personal and spiritual home study courses, with tutorial CDs, to support the seven spiritual openings. These courses are available as MP3 downloads – please view our website for where you can download them from. 'The Seekers Guide for a New Awakening' supporting courses are 'The Excellent You, 'Love and Relationships' and 'The Gateway to Enlightenment'.

When the CDs are listened to repeatedly, they have a transformative effect upon the consciousness of the listener. The 'Ah Ha' moments just keep coming over and over again. What could not be understood through reading alone becomes an enlightenment experience as the change in consciousness occurs at the soul level of awareness within you.

New Awakening teaches The Universal Life Healing Energy in three stages; Reiki 1st Degree, Reiki 2nd Degree, Reiki Master/Reiki Master Teacher, with each stage consisting of two parts. The first part is the professional home study multimedia course learning material. The second part is the practical 'Self Attunement' energy experience, that is provided free of charge, as our gift to you from our website. (www.new-awakening.co.uk)

About the Author

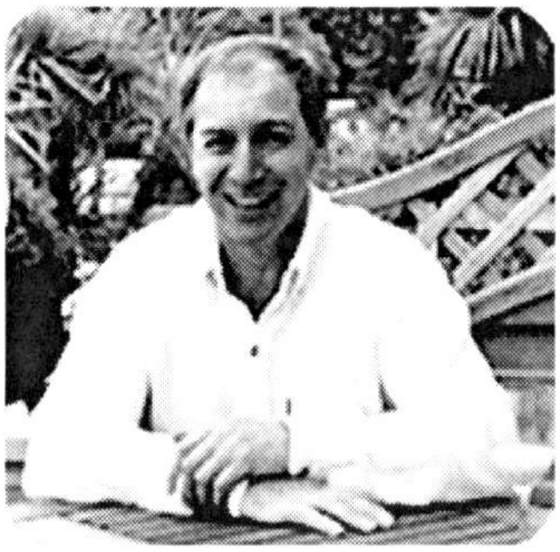

Robert Bourne is a Reiki Master Teacher, healer, author, resource manager for organisations and a spiritual course creator. He began his career in sports psychology, psychotherapy, hypnosis and NLP gaining an honours degree for his thesis on Auto-suggestion in 1986. In 1995 Spiritual fusion was experienced with the Beloved Universal Divine Consciousness revealing Robert's true mission as a spiritual teacher.

Robert was the founder of Reikiparty International, which was a friendship organisation uniting like-minded people. The Spiritual Organisation flowered in the spirit of Unconditional Love, whereby individuals who wished to unite with like minded friends were encouraged to do so by contacting each other with the view of helping and supporting each other on their spiritual journey. Reikiparty quickly evolved into a less structured organisation promoting the expanded spiritual system 'New Awakening'. This new spiritual holistic system is the compassionate flowering of the crown chakra within spiritual development. The organisation offers love, healing and friendship, providing guidance and encouragement for individuals who wish to hold fun events expressing the joy of Life. Because of the understanding that total freedom for the individual's personal expression of the Divine experience is embraced, no specific structure has been created as to how to hold events or support meetings. New Awakening supports those individuals who wish to make contact with other like minded friends in the form of providing 'how to do' free of charge downloads. You can find these free downloads from within our resource centre on our website at www.new-awakening.co.uk.

The expanded idea of the Reiki Healing Universal Life Energy being practiced for personal and spiritual development is now promoted to everyone. Reiki healing is seen as the first step to a greater energy experience of Unconditional Love to take place within the individual; to achieve an experience of bliss and Truth in the form of Divine wisdom and Oneness enlightenment.

It was in 2008 that the phenomenon of New-Awakening was created. This is an advanced energy training based upon an Unconditional Love energy transfer. The place where no conflict arises is the consciousness of Oneness, of Unity consciousness. It is this consciousness that is the foundation of this new people's organisation. It is this place where you will arrive through studying all four courses in this total system for spiritual enlightenment.

Robert, author and course creator for Naturally You Publishing, is currently living in Devon in the UK. Robert's life's purpose is to offer teachings and energy experiences to bring about a change in higher consciousness for the individual. The creation of value is always the first consideration when creating interactive courses. The vision is to create a golden age wherein society becomes a loving spiritual experience for the whole of mankind.

Finally Robert would like to share with you

"I am devoted to sharing the blissful
Divine connection of purity with you"

Namaste

Acknowledgments

I offer gratitude and appreciation to all my spiritual teachers, masters, friends, family and for their support and encouragement. Without the experience of meeting everyone in my life to date I would have never been able to have written this course. Thank you very much from the bottom of my heart to everyone I have ever met.

The following great people have helped me develop in knowledge, love and wisdom:

Osho – Bhagwan Shree Rajneesh, Amma and Bhagwan – Oneness movement, Deepak Chopra, Eckhart Tolle, Virginia Satir – family therapist and last but not least Deva Premal and Miten for their mystically uplifting music.

Caution and guidelines for your safety with Reiki

The exercises, hand positions and meditations described in this course manual are intended for the healing and harmonization of you as a holistic being. The course creator wishes to point out that, in the case of illness, a doctor or healing practitioner should always be consulted. The Reiki positions and meditations described may naturally be applied as an additional form of treatment. Reiki does not take the place of conventional medicine. Always consult your doctor for an acute or infectious condition and any problem of urgent concern.

Reiki is a complementary therapy that works effectively alongside orthodox and alternative health-care solutions.

Printed in the United Kingdom by
Lightning Source UK Ltd., Milton Keynes
140180UK00001B/3/P

9 780956 115928